234642 618

SPECIALIZED FUTURES

SPECIALIZED FUTURES

Essays in honour of

Sir George Godber GCB

IAN CRAFT, ERIC GAMBRILL
COLIN GODBER, DULCIE GOODING
MICHAEL GREEN, R. L. HIMSWORTH
TOM MEADE, ROSEMARY MULLIGAN
JEAN TURNER, PAUL VICKERS

Published for the
Nuffield Provincial Hospitals Trust
by the Oxford University Press
London New York Toronto
1975

Published for the
Nuffield Provincial Hospitals Trust
3 Prince Albert Road, London NW1 7SP
by the
Oxford University Press, Ely House, London W1

GLASGOW NEW YORK TORONTO MELBOURNE WELLINGTON
CAPE TOWN SALISBURY IBADAN NAIROBI DAR ES SALAAM LUSAKA ADDIS ABABA
BOMBAY CALCUTTA MADRAS KARACHI LAHORE DACCA
KUALA LUMPUR SINGAPORE HONG KONG TOKYO

ISBN 0 19 721388 X

Designed by Bernard Crossland
Printed in Great Britain by
Hazell Watson and Viney Ltd
Aylesbury, Bucks

Contents

Prefatory note

This collection is a tribute by the Trustees in honour of Sir George Godber who had an outstanding tenure as Chief Medical Officer of the DHSS from 1960 to 1973 and a long association with the Nuffield Provincial Hospitals Trust.

The latter in effect dates from the early years of the Trust's existence when it was engaged in a partnership from 1941 to 1945 with the then Ministry of Health to produce 'The Hospital Surveys' which were a Domesday Book of the hospitals as a necessary preliminary to their co-ordination in the Act of 1946.

Later on, when Sir George was Deputy CMO, he suggested and had the key role in the first of many policy seminars arranged by the Trust which was entitled 'Future Trends in Medicine'. If most of the participants at that small private meeting at Christ Church, Oxford, in 1957 were hardly unknown to the *cognoscenti*, they certainly had not become the luminaries in medicine they were later destined to be. Indeed the stimulation of fresh ideas from those with a future has long been a special characteristic of Sir George and he has constantly urged that opportunities be given to the young to express points of view which are not necessarily in tune with those of their elders.

The Trustees felt it would thus be appropriate to mark his retirement as well as adding to their own 'intelligence' by inviting him to nominate[1] a number of younger doctors who would be commissioned to write essays in which they would be asked to look ahead in their particular specialty and to speculate about its place within the NHS.

These essays were all written before the current crises in the NHS and while many of the issues touched upon in the essays are unlikely to be much affected by the crises, which sadly are more a reflection of the current uncertainties which run through so many sections of British society, it is only fair to the authors that this fact be noted.

January 1975 GORDON MCLACHLAN

1. In fact Sir George nominated all but one, the exception arising from editorial privilege in which I chose Dr Colin Godber. Ed.

Introduction

The long training period in medicine restricts in two ways the opportunities of younger doctors to express their views about the professional future which they rather than their mentors have to live. First the scientific and social content of learning medicine is absorbing in itself and leaves little time for the creation of the platform from which most people in the profession are heard, even if the young doctor has the urge to utter his views about organization. If he wants to write, it is likely to be on some scientific interest. Secondly the organization of the profession in Britain is in many ways hierarchical both in the NHS and in the powerful associations and colleges and there is no great incentive to the younger doctor, who may well be deeply involved in the pursuit of the memberships or fellowships virtually essential to his own professional advancement, to assert his views especially if they differ sharply from those of his senior colleagues. The deterrents operate at the local as well as at the national level. There are now channels through which the material interests of the younger doctors can be pressed, and very necessary they have proved to be, but only in psychiatry has there been a serious attempt to put forward the views of a younger group on other aspects of the future development of medicine or a part of it. Thirty-five years ago there was a group, Medical Planning Research, which formulated the views of younger doctors on health service needs, but it had no successors.

The BMA, the Royal Colleges, and the specialty associations all have their own ways of allowing the ventilation of views of those of their members who qualified recently to be heard, but the voices are somewhat muted in the more assured collective utterances of these bodies. This is especially true in regard to new developments in the NHS. One need only look back on the struggles of specialties now recognized to emerge from the over-possessive embrace of the established specialties like general medicine and general surgery to appreciate how conservative the profession can be. Twenty-five years ago some orthopaedic surgeons and chest physicians were stoutly maintaining that they had no need for a radiologist's opinion on the films taken of their patients, and most English regions were quite unready for the development of departments of urology. Much later than that cardio-respiratory investigation was often held to be a proper activity for a senior registrar who would have no future outlet, rather than for a consultant in clinical physiology—even though there were by then eight chairs in this specialty in Sweden.

As one who had tried to find opportunities of learning what younger doctors thought, even from the fastnesses of the Elephant and Castle, I therefore welcomed this initiative of the NPHT in offering to a small group of doctors, all qualified after the first decade of the NHS, the opportunity to write about the future for their own branches of medicine and in some ways about the future developments in health care. It was a particular privilege to be given the opportunity of choosing all but one of the ten invited. They were all people with whom I had had some contact and their essays show that each of them has a fresh approach to a part of the future of medicine. The essays were not prepared to any agreed structure although most of the authors met on two occasions. No attempt was made to secure uniformity of views, and indeed some sharp differences appear. Nor did Mr McLachlan or I do more than suggest some minor points of fact—not opinion—which might not have been available to the individual when he or she was writing the essay. In that sense this collection of essays is unedited.

Despite the different paths the authors have followed there is neither irreconcilable divergence nor great overlap between the contributions. Each is well worth reading for its own sake and collectively they contain promise for the future of British medicine which is reassuring against the background of the present conflicts. It would have been interesting to include similar contributions from members of the other health professions, but that would have been less easily arranged and a large increase in bulk would have been needed. This, after all, is about the future of medicine within the NHS rather than the NHS itself. At the time of writing there is great dissension within the NHS and the family of the health professions is divided within itself. Those divisions arise mainly from the knowledge of all working in the NHS that the resources available to it are insufficient. Everyone knows that the capability of medicine (using that term to include not only the work of doctors but also of all those who work with them) exceeds the resources available. Medicine in this sense is an open-ended commitment, and no country will ever be able to provide for all that could conceivably be done. But it is widely believed within the service that it has been progressively starved to the point where there is no longer enough to keep the central core of the service at the level of efficiency which makes it possible to do the best with what we have. Moreover, there is inequality in distribution which means that some regions fall behind the rest. Perhaps some of the shortfall could be met by greater efficiency or better choice of priorities.

Strikingly none of these essays wastes the opportunity of discussing truly professional problems by digressing into the medico-political field. Paul Vickers has commented on some of the financial problems along with a discussion of the very difficult issues of accident and emergency work and medical career development in hospital. His views on medical administration are those of one who once contemplated such a career and link with the discussion by Dulcie Gooding of the development of community medicine as a specialty. This development is one of great interest to other countries and to the World Health Organization because it is being deliberately fostered to a greater extent than elsewhere. Richard Himsworth has written from the background of the clinical research centre not only on hospital medicine but also with an appreciation of its dependence on the growing strength of general practice which older 'specialists' do not always show. Rosemary Mulligan not only expresses her views on the development of chest medicine but also demonstrates the level of professional satisfaction which the doctor trained in the relatively affluent circumstances of London teaching hospitals can find in the district partnership with general practice and specialist colleagues which is much more readily attained in the real England outside the great cities. Michael Green and Colin Godber have contributed companion pieces on the two greatest problems of the NHS, the care of long-stay patients whether mentally ill or retarded or suffering chronic physical illness. They bring out very clearly the dependence of these services on close working with the personal social services of local authorities and the need to encourage the parallel development of those services. Jean Turner has found time, despite her imminent departure to work in Iran, to write a most interesting commentary on the relationship between general surgery and the surgical specialties. One hopes that this reflects a greater readiness among young surgeons now to recognize the need for specialization than was present twenty years ago. Eric Gambrill has written one of the best short descriptions of the kind of general practice we are seeking to achieve. The NHS in allowing British general practice to evolve in the form now to be seen in the best conditions has made it possible for us to have the best primary care system in any country. That may have happened more by good fortune than original design but it has certainly been deliberately encouraged in later years. Ian Craft describes changes in both obstetrics and gynaecology which are already in progress and points to the need for better evaluation of results which Tom Meade develops in his chapter on epidemiology. The quotation from Lord Rosenheim with which that chapter begins could be the text for the whole volume. The NHS moves steadily further along a road which leads to better service both curative and preventive for every district. We need the evaluation of district services which the epidemiologist and community physician can combine to give, but also to retain the personal relationship with the individual patient which every good doctor must have as his guide in his daily work. A specialty missing from the collection is pathology only because the review which was commissioned has not come to hand. This is unfortunate because it is one of the most difficult areas in which expansion is continuous and rapid and threatens to swamp the clinician with the sheer volume of the information he himself requests from the laboratory. Not only more careful selection but also some simplifying mechanism to help comprehension of this mass of information will be necessary if expansion continues. Fortunately the right of the GP to a direct service is no longer contested, but we still lack sound apparatus for use in the course of primary care. Paradoxically one of the great threats to the budget of the NHS could be multiplication of 'office-use' systems of uncertain comparability.

Finally I will quote the last paragraph of the Michael M. Davis Lecture given in Chicago in 1969.[1]

I end with a quotation from the New England Medical Journal published just eight weeks ago. 'Medical care is increasingly fragmented and complex, and the warmth of a long term association with a single physician has become a luxury for a few rather than the customary setting for the delivery of health care.'[2] I do not know if that is true here. I do know that it is our wish and intention that it shall not be true in Britain.

GEORGE GODBER

1. Godber, Sir George, *The Future Place of the Personal Physician,* Michael M. Davis Lecture (University of Chicago, 1969).
2. Francis, V., Korsch, B. M., and Morris, M. J., 'Gaps in doctor–patient communications', *New Engl. Med. J.* (March 1969), p. 535.

Orthopaedics

PAUL VICKERS

PAUL VICKERS
MA, FRCS.Ed, FRCSE
Orthopaedic Surgeon

Orthopaedics

Like my fellow contributors to this book, I have been given a great deal of latitude in my subject matter. I propose to discuss five separate topics which are of interest to me. I start by discussing the provision of comprehensive health care systems.

John Locke believed that all men were equal and independent. The ideal of the NHS was to enable the very best in health care to be available to all. This is not the same quality of equality that John Locke was discussing. At the inception of the NHS it was believed that, if a comprehensive health care system were provided, the population would enjoy better health and the demands on the service and therefore its cost would fall. Unfortunately, the early planners had miscalculated in both the fact that new frontiers in the fight against disease would constantly become surmountable (often expensively) and, secondly, in the fact that, in overcoming a disease, we tend to upset a natural balance about which we know little, and the defeated disease or another tends to return, often in a more insidious and dangerous form.

Given unlimited funds and manpower, many diseases could be overcome for a population. Unfortunately, the NHS does not have unlimited funds, for the Secretary of State, acting on the advice of his officers at the DHSS, has to argue his case with the Treasury. Funding is therefore finite and, indeed, were this not so, the taxpayers of this country (and all who live in this country pay taxes, either directly or indirectly) would soon express their displeasure. The medical administrators are therefore one of several groups who have to make value judgements between the patient on the one hand and a limited budget on the other.

The medical administrator occupies the difficult position between the administrators, whose natural emphasis is on the organization of a smooth-running health care system, and the clinician, whose prime interest must always be to look after his particular patients and to press for more resources for his particular interest. It would be wrong for a clinician not to express himself strongly on these matters. On the other hand, the medical administrator has to attempt to make value judgements to identify areas of need and to correct imbalances, for (as is the case in most of man's activities) the largest numbers with the loudest voice tend to be served with the biggest slice of the cake; this is not always just.

In theory, the NHS should allocate resources to the areas of greatest need. Again, in theory, these areas of need should coincide with areas giving the greatest economic benefit to the nation. I am sure that the most frustrating part of a medical administrator's life is that he can take an over-all view of the service and can identify areas of need and of potential economic benefit, but he has to act on advice which represents a great many differing interests. The number of doctors with an extensive knowledge of medicine outside their own field is not large. Individual specialties tend to group professionally and socially together, and one learns about the problems in other fields only by meeting practitioners in those fields professionally and socially.

The division of the profession into three groups in 1948 was one of the biggest difficulties in the old health service. Before this time there had been much more contact and exchange of information between the hospital side of the profession and general practice. Indeed, many doctors practised with distinction simultaneously in both fields. After 1948, this became much more difficult. I hope that 1974 will make it easier again, for it is essential for the profession to speak with one voice, especially if value judgements are to be made. Over the past ten years there has been some tendency for GPs to undertake part-time posts in hospitals more frequently; this has been possible because of their more limited contract. Interest in the other direction has been largely limited to junior hospital staff undertaking emergency call duties and locum work. It is difficult for either a whole-time or a maximum part-time consultant to devote any significant part of his time to general practice owing to the limitations imposed by contract.

Medical care has always been expensive and beyond the reach of many, for purely financial reasons. It was hoped that the NHS would eliminate this financial barrier. It is difficult to argue that any inhabitant of this country is more or less deserving because of the area where he resides. Yet, with the vastly increasing cost of health care, to which I can see no end, a financial limitation on the availability of health care is again in operation. Whereas formerly it was the expense the individual could afford, now it is the expense the country is willing to afford. Moreover, in health care terms, the citizens of this country are not equal. The original lack of equality of the NHS in 1948 was perpetuated by percentage increases in budgets. The effect of this, coupled with inflation, was to make rich areas richer, whilst poor areas became poorer. Irrespective of the skill of doctors and ancillary staffs, manpower and facilities are most unevenly distributed. Rich hospitals and areas defend their position as being centres of excellence, forgetting the corollary of their claims. To some extent, the financial structuring of the new Health Service may help to even out these disparities, but they are truly very gross.

The greatest difficulty in the new Health Service, from the clinicians' point of view, is the immense amount of time which it requires of them for administrative duties. Doctors enter clinical practice because it is what they wish to do, not because they wish to sit on committees and, because they are not trained in administration, they regard this type of activity as a double waste of time. It is essential, however, for all doctors to be as aware of current organization as of current clinical practice and to be lacking in knowledge of one field is as dangerous as to be lacking in knowledge of the other. If doctors do not take an active part, they may well, by default, be party to decisions they oppose. This is the cleft stick in which the profession finds itself today. The most important decisions involve the allocation of limited resources. Should a particular area have an intensive care unit, a dialysis unit, or a geriatric day-hospital or even worse, which unit should be closed? I doubt if any member of the profession would enjoy being party to these decisions, which relate intimately to the well-being or otherwise of their patients. When these decisions have to be made, as I feel they will, the profession will have to make it very clear that the restriction on services is not imposed by and, indeed, is not the wish of the profession.

In the present economic climate, meaningful discussion on the cost of health care is very difficult. So many of the drugs and so much of the equipment which doctors in and out of hospital have come to use every day are increasing enormously in cost. This inflation will give rise to further restrictions on the purchasing power of budgets. The unpalatable truth is that, whereas we as a profession would wish to provide the best possible health care for all in need of it, health care costs money, and this money is paid by the patient or those who may become patients. This is just as true of our National Health Service as in other health care systems. The only difference is in the method of finance, the enormous cost of health care in this country being borne by direct and indirect taxation.

It is naturally in the interests of all that health care be administered as economically as possible, but a decision to limit health care on the grounds of cost is one the profession must avoid. The DHSS has only made such a recommendation directly in the context of heart transplants but, indirectly, this decision is made every day. I believe that efficient health care may be of financial benefit to the State, as when a total hip replacement enables a solitary, elderly lady to look after herself, avoiding the cost of living in an institution, as a bonus on top of improving her quality of life. Again, efficient primary treatment of a minor hand injury may save a young person from weeks of disability, with consequent economic loss both to the individual and to the State.

It is always worth experimenting in cutting costs and, indeed, several such experiments are in progress, increasing the scope of out-patient surgery or planning a procedure, to take place in the course of a Monday to Friday admission. One must be wary with these procedures, however, lest they merely transfer an expense from one ledger to another. The same is true of experiments to make more efficient use of expensive apparatus by shift working. Some patients may, indeed, find it more convenient to attend for investigation outside normal working hours, but this type of work would undoubtedly be inconvenient for doctors and the essential technicians. Furthermore, one must remember that complex equipment needs to be maintained. For instance, operating theatres which are over-used tend to be under-cleaned, and the rate of infection increases. The difficulty with the NHS is that it gives the doctor an open-ended commitment which, for reasons beyond his control, he is unable to meet.

The other great difficulty for the profession in the NHS is the relationship between the ratio of GPs and consultants to junior hospital staff. This was a difficulty which was created in 1948 and has led to a situation where today 4,500 junior staff are required to fill expected vacancies both in general practice and among hospital consultants. There are approximately 25,000 established principals in general practice and 12,000 consultants in the NHS, assuming three years' training for general practice and ten years' training for a hospital specialty, we cannot justify more than 5,000 junior staff. In fact, we have nearly 20,000 junior hospital staff, approximately half of whom come from overseas. Even if all the doctors from overseas returned home, and it is claimed that this would cause the NHS to collapse, it is difficult to see what the future holds for many of the graduates of this country. This is a problem the profession must solve. It is almost unique to this country. Perhaps we have geared the consultant too low or, alternatively, too high. In few other countries does every doctor acting in the 'consultant' role expect a retinue of junior staff. Yet all these younger doctors believe themselves to be in training for something, and are encouraged in this belief. This is immoral.

The only control over junior staff numbers has been at senior registrar level, the numbers of senior registrars being geared approximately to expected consultant vacancies. Senior registrar posts are held overwhelmingly in teaching centres. Recently the position has been complicated by the recognition, for the purpose of specialist accreditation, of certain registrar posts. Although most senior registrars in this country can expect to become consultants, most consultant posts are in district hospitals. The conditions of work are so different in district hospitals, as compared with teaching hospitals where most senior registrars are trained, that the purely teaching hospital trained senior registrar is ill-equipped to carry out his work in a district hospital, and I could quote instances where he does it badly. The accusation is made that in district hospitals a senior registrar is used as a 'pair of hands'; this was certainly not my experience. I found myself to be *the* senior registrar in a district general hospital and was carefully supervised and conscientiously instructed, unlike some of my colleagues in teaching hospitals. I should not wish to abolish a teaching hospital component, but I would hope that all posts at this level would include an effective rotation. It is unfortunate that posts being recognized for specialist accreditation appear to be strongly teaching hospital orientated. This is curiously similar to the pattern of training which hitherto existed in France.

A further major problem on the hospital side of the profession is 'shortage specialties'. These are specialties which few doctors wish to enter. I believe that the three major specialties have an unwarranted influence on undergraduate teaching. There are so many different satisfying ways of practising medicine; yet most undergraduates are made to feel that if they do not achieve a consultant post in one of the three major specialties they will have failed. This is manifestly untrue, and the only way around this difficulty that I can see is to increase the exposure to shortage specialties in the undergraduate and immediate postgraduate years. There is certainly much more room for positive career counselling in medicine. It is interesting that in the specialty of pathology the one subspecialty to which there is good exposure as an undergraduate is morbid anatomy, in this specialty there are good fields of recruitment.

Finally, in this section it is important to realize that, in a situation where resources for funding the service will always be limited, the profession will be faced with the choice as to whether it wishes to provide a particular service, carry out a piece of research, or to receive higher incomes. The opportunities for dividing the profession against itself in this way are many. A divided profession will undoubtedly find that its socio-economic standing falls. I believe that standards of practice may, in fact, also fall if this happens.

The clinical subject in which I received most of my training was orthopaedic surgery. The two fundamental divisions in orthopaedic surgery, the surgery of trauma and elective surgery, have given rise to much unease. Are they in fact separate, or are they related? The management of accident or war injury must have been one of the earliest medical preoccupations of man, and it is interesting to speculate whether it may not indeed predate internal medicine. I am fortunate enough to own a 1657 edition of *De Medicina* by A. Cornelius Celsus, published by Elsevier Press. The chapter 'De Fractura Femora' would be understood easily by any orthopaedic surgeon today. It is also interesting to speculate as to how many of today's massive output of textbooks will survive the fifteen hundred years for which this book was a standard medical textbook.

Most pre-Listerian surgery was peripheral surgery and therefore of an orthopaedic nature and, to this extent, orthopaedic surgeons can claim to be the true descendants of earlier surgeons, with much more validity than can today's general surgeons. Accounts of early surgery, even at the hands of masters such as Dupuytren at the 'Hotel Dieu', are horrific and the mortality, from what were obviously tetanus and streptococcal infection, ran at around 75 per cent. The other root of orthopaedic surgery lay in the 'bone setters', and it is interesting that these are still to be found in the 'yellow pages' of our telephone directories today. These two roots of orthopaedic surgery were brought together by men such as Hugh Owen Thomas and Robert Jones to establish the specialty as we know it today.

The early orthopaedic surgeons were concerned with the management and treatment of trauma, especially fractures, acute and chronic infection (notably chronic osteomyelitis and tuberculosis) and in the correction of congenital and acquired deformities. The risk of formal corrective operations on bone could only be taken after Lister had established antisepsis. McEwen had encouraged asepsis, and adequate anaesthesia was available.

The major crippling diseases before and after the Second World War were tuberculosis and poliomyelitis, the conquest of rickets having become possible somewhat earlier. It was thought that, with the conquest of these diseases, there was but a limited future for orthopaedic surgery. This was the background behind the suggestion that orthopaedic surgeons should have control of accident departments. In fact, things have turned out very differently. Orthopaedic surgeons have found that they have an important role to play in the management of both rheumatoid and osteo-arthrosis and, in addition, advances in paediatrics and neurosurgery have ensured the survival of many children with congenital deformities who would formerly have died. Many of these require multiple corrective operations, and much in the way of appliances and equipment. As if this were not enough, the old enemies, rickets and tuberculosis, are again making their appearance, especially in immigrant communities, and infection in the shape of staphylococci and pseudomonas are the constant concern of all who carry out major operations on bones. Truly, the field of orthopaedic surgery is now so vast that it is difficult for one man to be a master of it all and already the tendency to specialize within the specialty is well established. I believe that the situation has become so complex that the time has come for the establishment of subspecialties.

Does orthopaedic surgery today justify itself in the terms I considered in the first part of this essay? The answer to this is, I feel, an only slightly qualified 'Yes'. The surgery of arthritis is an immensely rewarding field. Total hip replacement, although an expensive procedure, must have improved the quality of life of many thousands of patients, enabling them to live independent and often economically productive lives, in addition to saving the State the cost of the institutional care which might well have been necessary otherwise. Similarly, surgery of the metacarpo-phalangeal joints of the hand has been a great boon to many, and the surgery of other joints a help to some. One must, however, remember that all is not credit. There are a substantial number of disasters, resulting from joint replacement surgery. Often these disasters have been due to attempts to treat a diseased joint, rather than a disease or a patient. This type of surgery is a field where a physician and a surgeon should treat a patient together. One reason for this is that some surgeons tend to be extroverted and under-critical; another is the complexity of the modern drug treatment for arthritis. Arthritis of both major types should be managed by a team, who together consider the place for medication, physiotherapy, and surgery. In terms of economic returns to the country, the benefit of orthopaedic surgery in this field is immense. It may truly be said that the country cannot afford not to maintain these services.

The surgery of multiple deformities, such as those associated with spina bifida is, however, much less rewarding. In some cases there is probably some improvement in the quality of life of an individual but in many ways the surgeon is providing psychiatric treatment in the form of hope for the parents of these children and eventually this may fail to be succeeded by despair. The maintenance of these children involves the support of their family unit, and the orthopaedic surgeon may fail even in this. So often a whole series of major operative procedures may be undertaken on a child of poor physique and limited intelligence for an end result which must be considered good, if it is marginally better than the original state. These major problems are not of the orthopaedic surgeons' creation. I feel that, if we are to continue with the present policy of preserving life for its own sake, without considering its quality (and we may be on dangerous ground if we do not), it is only fair that this burden, which has fallen upon the orthopaedic surgeons, should be shared with paediatricians, and later, with some category of interested physicians. This is not to say that this field of surgery is not, on occasion, very rewarding. There are some children for whom a great deal can be done, and results can be most gratifying. In terms of economic returns to the nation, however, this balance sheet will never be in credit. Personally, I believe strongly that the argument that this field of surgery is justified on the grounds of the advances it may produce is immoral. If we regard these children as human beings, then it is wrong to experiment on them. I find the whole field of multiple operations and extensive supporting apparatus most depressing.

The management of other congenital abnormalities, such as talipes, congenital dislocation of the hip and even scoliosis, however, is undoubtedly a most rewarding and worthwhile field; worthwhile in getting to know a child as he or she grows, and worthwhile in the terms that a disability can often be corrected and overcome. Here is a field where the doctor–patient–parent relationship is at its most personal and rewarding. Again, besides being rewarding on a personal level, the returns to the community are high. This is immensely worthwhile work, and work which merits further research and development. The paediatric orthopaedic surgeon can therefore find his work most rewarding.

The complaint of most orthopaedic surgeons is the problem of managing fractured necks of femur in elderly ladies. This is a high-risk group of patients and, when an orthopaedic surgeon attempts to achieve early mobilization of a patient by early operation which may offer the best chance of life to that patient, he is undertaking a major procedure on a patient who, if she suffered a comparable medical illness (say, a coronary thrombosis or a stroke), would receive maintenance treatment only from physicians, to be followed by our grossly inadequate rehabilitation facilities. It is hardly surprising that many of these patients die before, during, or after surgery. When the operation is successful, the orthopaedic surgeon knows that his problems have only just begun, and the likelihood is that the lady will be single and live alone (perhaps these were factors in the aetiology of the original fracture). Often rehabilitation is slow, and a return to the conditions from which the patient was admitted may be socially unacceptable. There is often a feeling on the part of the surgeon that he has not done much good, either to the patient or to society, and this may be aggravated by the fact that the patient is occupying a bed which the surgeon, faced with a waiting-list for routine orthopaedic surgery, feels he could put to better use. The social services, however, tend to regard the fact that the patient is in a bed in hospital as indicating that the problem is not urgent. They forget that hospital resources are limited, and efficiency depends on maintaining a turnover; blocked beds benefit no-one and, in fact, often least of all the social services themselves. There is an urgent need for more sheltered accommodation with some supportive services, such as physiotherapy and occupational therapy, through which these patients may pass during their return to their home environments. There is also a need for day-hospital accommodation for this type of patient, and such provision would enable many relatives to support patients who would otherwise need to be in an institution. The great problem, however, as the orthopaedic surgeon sees it, is in the efficient use of orthopaedic beds.

Another field of orthopaedics is an old one, the management of fractures. Most fractures require regular review to check position, check plaster, and to keep an eye on and advise the patient. By and large, the general public has a very poor idea of the duration of disability to be expected from a fracture, and we must be ready to volunteer this advice in a humane way. The difficulties with fracture clinics in which a large number of patients are seen are the difficulties in establishing a rapport with patients quickly, in anticipating what may go wrong and in the question of deciding when an operation is indicated. I feel strongly that properly supervised fracture clinics are the best way of managing these injuries. The same is true of hand injuries. In some centres, hands are not dealt with by an orthopaedic surgeon. This does not matter, as the principle is that of regular supervision. A badly managed hand injury can result in prolonged, unnecessary disability, and properly supervised hand clinics are the best insurance against this. Both fracture clinics and hand clinics form essential parts of health care systems, being immensely worthwhile to both the individual and the community. Improperly supervised clinics are as bad, if not worse, than faulty insurance policies, as they share with such policies the generation of a dangerous and false sense of security.

Orthopaedic surgery has tended to fail in one field, that of undergraduate education. This is reflected in a lack of knowledge of orthopaedics among GPs and others practising in different fields. This leads to misunderstandings and, in fact, to an extra workload on orthopaedic surgeons. This form of mystique is most unfortunate in any specialty.

I hope I have justified orthopaedic surgery, and indicated the areas where advances are needed or, indeed, where I would hope they will be made. I feel that orthopaedic surgery is immensely worthwhile as a career and, in more mundane terms, as an investment for the nation. I have only one reservation and that is the high cost of orthopaedic instruments and apparatus. To some extent, it might be possible to mitigate this by establishing regional 'banks' of instruments, from which the instruments for a particular operation could be borrowed when required. Many instruments are, in fact, used only rarely, and represent a waste of capital while they lie unused on theatre shelves. At the same time, the facilities available to any individual surgeon would be widened.

The future of orthopaedics lies, as with so many other branches of medicine, in increasing specialization, associated with increased experience and, I would hope, consequent increased skill of the practitioner. This is obviously a good thing, but such 'super-specialists' must always remember that they do not treat diseases, but rather patients as a whole. It is a disaster for a patient to come under the care of the wrong super-specialist. If the tendency to super-specialization is to continue it is only tolerable if it is associated with a very high standard of general practice.

The third subject is the running and function of casualty departments. In the second part of this essay, I mentioned the reasons why many casualty departments have been administered by orthopaedic surgeons and the reasons why orthopaedic surgeons often found it difficult to carry out these functions: they just could not spare the time. The same consideration also applied to consultants in other specialties, who were appointed to take charge of casualty departments. This situation was aggravated by the fact that, once the war-trained consultants had become more senior, their successors in charge of casualty departments tended to have little training for the job and, in any case, it was not what they wished to do. The scene was, in fact, set for the establishment of a new specialty. It is possible that the happiest way this could have been achieved may have been as a subspecialty of orthopaedics, but this proved impossible because of numerous fears felt by orthopaedic surgeons over the possible loss of control over the important initial treatment of fractures, and also because orthopaedic departments had become dependent for junior hospital staff on the fact that a period of six months' 'training in casualty' had been made mandatory for all candidates taking the Final English FRCS. This last decision was, in my opinion, a disaster, since it provided a captive labour force and so countered pressures, which would otherwise have forced the casualty crisis into the open at a much earlier date. I believe that improvement in the educational content of casualty posts and in the standards of work done would have been made long ago, but for this decision.

Of course, orthopaedics forms only a small percentage of the casualty workload. Many other specialties are involved. It could be argued that practitioners in all specialties, including general practice, would benefit from a period of training in casualty, but I do not believe that the Royal College of General Practitioners, or any other College supervising postgraduate training, will allow its trainees into casualty posts unless it has first ensured that training will be given.

An organization which has a major interest in casualty departments and the specialty of casualty medicine is the body at present known as 'The Casualty Surgeons' Association'. This organization was founded by a group of senior casualty officers, who in fact had acted as casualty consultants for many years. More recently, the Bruce Committee recommended the appointment of a number of consultants in casualty medicine. This number, at the time of writing, is approaching one hundred, which makes it a larger specialty than many of those which are already established. The two difficulties are that this specialty still lacks a recognized training programme, and it has yet to establish the parameters of its work, though the broad interests and lack of boundaries will be welcomed by many.

More than any other department of a hospital, the casualty department can claim to be the most important. Here the two great branches of the profession are in daily if, unfortunately, often indirect contact. Here the hospital, as opposed to the GP, is in daily contact with the public. Here the complex structure of the hospital service must show that the individuals who are doctors and nurses chose their profession to serve and to be kind to patients.

The former practice of appointing a junior general, or orthopaedic consultant to take charge of a casualty department, with a view to 'promotion' later, had some successes, and many eminent surgeons have reached the top of their field by this ladder. It is not so readily accepted that the system also enabled the less competent to achieve a certain elevation and importance. The system was, however, appalling for the casualty departments. No doctor could run a casualty department if he were constantly guarding his future prospects for promotion; besides which, it is impossible to argue that being a consultant in charge of a casualty department is a suitable training or even a suitable holding post for a future consultant in general or orthopaedic surgery. Casualty departments can only receive the care and supervision they require if they are run by consultants who are fully committed to them. The arguments against the specialty are first, the lack of continuity of patient care. This argument could also be levelled against the large specialties of anaesthetics and pathology, and is invalid. Any consultant is at liberty to follow up his own special interests in his field and, in casualty, the field is wide open. The second argument is that no-one worthwhile would enter this field because it is not rewarding. This argument is about as valid as an orthopaedic surgeon saying that he does not know why people wish to carry out prostatectomies.

Staffing at a senior level in casualty departments is related to staffing at junior levels for, until adequate instruction and supervision are given, the junior casualty officer's job cannot be made worthwhile. It is immoral to force junior staff into unrewarding posts by rotation and training schemes, when no training is given. The duties of the consultant in casualty medicine are to teach and supervise the junior staff in the department (surely worthwhile in itself), to establish the parameters of work to be done in the department (by liaison with the public, GPs, and other hospital departments), to establish a workable major accident scheme and to follow trends in casualty attendances. The casualty consultant must have a wide experience, and be able to make decisions quickly. He should be able to cover a wide field with considerable competence, being able and willing to ask and receive help when he needs it. This implies the difficult capacity for self-criticism.

There are two fundamental and interrelated questions: 'What kind of work do we wish our casualty departments to do?' and 'Whom do we wish to be in charge?'. The workload in casualty is very variable in type and quantity. Even if we confine our discussion to trauma, patterns of trauma differ from department to department and, in many departments in fact, trauma forms only a minor part of the workload, the remainder being made up of the acute medical and surgical conditions, the inescapable problem of the casual attender and referrals from general practice. It is to be hoped that the further opinion obtained will be better than that of an inadequately trained and supervised casualty officer, who has been used in this way so often in the past.

Casual attenders present special problems. They may represent underlying social and psychological stresses which hitherto we have failed to recognize. These patients may well need our help, but often not in the way they ask for it. They are often an unpleasant, litigious, and distasteful group to deal with, and they occupy much of a casualty officer's time. Many of them attend because they know that they would get 'short shrift' from their GPs and yet the casualty officer has to examine them in case they are physically ill. This is an area where communication between GP and casualty department is essential. There may be situations where we can help but undoubtedly these patients would be better handled by their GP, who knows them and who can claim a measure of authority over them, which the young and inexperienced casualty officer cannot do.

The efficient running of a casualty department depends upon organizing liaison between the many different interests involved. A further strong argument in favour of this specialty is the difficulty a specialist has in assessing conditions outside his field.

Someone is needed who can take an over-all view of, say, a patient with multiple trauma, and this should be one of the duties of the casualty consultant. It seems likely that the basic mechanism involved in shock, whether of surgical or medical origin, are similar, and that the management of the various forms of shock is interrelated. It therefore seems reasonable for consultants in casualty medicine to have an interest in intensive care and the problems of shock.

As I stated in the first section, economic factors are influencing our practice of medicine. It is to be hoped that by competent supervision of minor injuries, casualty consultants would ensure that such injuries do not lead to major economic loss to the individual and the community, as has so often happened in the past. It is also to be hoped that a properly established department would, in fact, save money and staff. If a department were to be provided with admission wards, in many hospitals this would reduce the demands on other individual departments which have to be staffed to the level required to receive emergencies. This need not deprive the present specialties of their interests or patients, but could be part of progressive patient care. There would also be no further need for undignified arguments as to which specialty a patient should be treated under.

It would seem therefore that: (1) the casualty consultant should have a working knowledge of several specialties, not to practise as a specialist in these fields, but rather to enable him to work in co-operation with the established specialisms. (2) This consultant should function in the 'primary physician' role, with the support of sophisticated techniques provided by the hospital. (3) He must be able to co-operate with his hospital colleagues, GPs, and with the social services. (4) He must not be placed in the position where he is undertaking the work of any other hospital specialty or of GPs. (5) This consultant must be, principally, a person who can take decisions rapidly. (6) His likely clinical responsibilities will include resuscitation and triage.

The training programme for this specialty must be designed to enhance decision-taking and leadership. It must be flexible enough to allow for gaps in a trainee's knowledge to be filled (for example, a surgically orientated trainee may require experience in cardiac intensive care, toxicology, and paediatrics). It is a personal view that the most likely field of recruitment is to be found among those younger doctors who have recently obtained the FRCS or MRCP. Although the position is changing, traditionally a surgeon has to make rapid decisions whether these be correct or not. In truth, this is a marvellous specialty to enter, for any doctor entering it now has freedom to employ his talents as he wishes; he is at liberty to follow special interests, and the job is really what he makes of it. I know of no other field of medicine where the opportunities, the need, and the potential satisfaction are so great. Casualty is an area of activity where the country must invest more funds, as the returns would be both substantial and easy to establish. The consultant in casualty medicine is a co-ordinator with a wide interest involving many different aspects of health care or in other words several different health care teams.

Having discussed one of the Cinderellas of medicine, I should now like to discuss another: rehabilitation. Again, because many different interests are involved, rehabilitation is a difficult subject to define. It is generally believed that many illnesses involve an acute period followed by a period of convalescence, after which the individual returns to his or her former level of activity. Of course, this is only true to a limited extent. Many illnesses, in fact, lead to varying degrees of disability of varying degrees of permanence. It is unfortunate that the National Insurance sickness scheme and, indeed, many private sickness schemes are phrased in terms which allow an individual to be either well or sick, with no allowance for the intermediate period, through which all who become sick must pass.

The objectives of rehabilitation also change with age. To a considerable degree the young can rehabilitate themselves and it is only when they are severely handicapped by injury or congenital abnormality that rehabilitation services are required to any extent. During the years of maturity rehabilitation is aimed at returning the individual to his or her optimal place in work and society and this is an objective which is worthy of intensive activity from all those who are involved in the rehabilitation field. The same objectives are true of the elderly but here the pace is somewhat slower, but we must not return to the former state when the illnesses and the infirmities of old age were regarded with complacence; here much can be done but progress generally is slower and it requires a more patient approach.

The concept of rehabilitation is a difficult one. Like so many developments in medicine, it was advanced rapidly along a narrow path under the stimulus of war. The stimulus in the last war was to get trained soldiers, sailors, and aircrew back into action as quickly as possible following physical injury. To this end, the various arms of the Forces developed their individual rehabilitation services; the coal industry (which suffered a similar shortage of trained manpower) developed a similar system. The aim of these rehabilitation centres was to return a trained man, following physical injury, to his former level of activity. This was not always possible, and the secondary objective became clear, which was to return the patient to the highest level of activity to which he was capable. The secondary objective opened the concept of rehabilitation to possible application to a whole range of diseases, complete recovery from which could not be anticipated or would be long delayed. Many of those involved in rehabilitation during the war regret this broadening of interest, claiming, with considerable justification, that rehabilitation for patients who have been psychiatrically or medically ill must be different in quality and quantity from that which was devised to deal with physical injury.

Whilst not questioning the fact that rehabilitation is a wide problem involving many different disciplines, I doubt if the medical rehabilitation centre (with its hard and long day of physical education, gymnastics, occupational therapy, assault courses, and work geared to future employment) is feasible for the rehabilitation of all illness for which rehabilitation is required. The rehabilitation centres, as envisaged in the new district general hospitals, will not be able to provide the duration, scope, or intensity of activity which was a part of the pattern of life in the rehabilitation centres. They are not large enough, and the needs of the differing patients will vary so much. I doubt whether the same quality of result will be obtained.

To some extent, the problem is not dissimilar to that of a casualty department in reverse. A casualty department receives, sorts, and distributes to a wide variety of points. It is to be expected that rehabilitation will receive, from a wide variety of points, patients at varying levels of activity and return them to the community at the highest level of activity which the centre can achieve. I feel that there is considerable danger that this level of activity will not be the highest possible attainable by that patient. There is the added difficulty of medical staff. Rehabilitation tends to come under the administration of a rheumatologist, or of an orthopaedic surgeon. By and large, it is rarely the major interest of this doctor and, whereas rehabilitation in their respective specialties is of interest to each, in few instances can either be expected to be knowledgeable beyond their own field.

The profession, as represented by all the various specialists who might conceivably have an interest in rehabilitation, must decide whether it wishes individual interests in rehabilitation to be sublimated to a rehabilitation centre. This might be relatively easy but, when there is considerable uncertainty as to the quality of the end-product of this new concept of rehabilitation, many doctors will have misgivings. To put the difficulty another way, there is undoubtedly a need for rehabilitation in many fields, but it does not follow that the rehabilitation required is always the same, or that the needs can be met in the same or even a similar way.

As with casualty, there is also the problem of who is to take charge. There is very little training in rehabilitation in this country, apart from that at the spinal injuries centres, and there is no training in the context of centres dealing with all forms of rehabilitation. In casualty there was a reservoir of likely applicants for the posts of casualty consultants, but there does not appear to be any corresponding reserve of likely applicants for consultants in rehabilitation. I feel that there will be considerable difficulty in filling any more than a handful of these posts. A further difficulty which is clear to me, having trained in orthopaedic surgery (and which I have no doubt is also true in other specialties, if in a different way), is that a good operation may be ruined by indifferent after-care; just as good after-care can can make a success of a less than perfectly performed operation. If rehabilitation centres, as planned, are to be staffed by rehabilitation specialists, then referring specialists will need to have great faith in them. Such faith can only develop over many years, and this is where the idea of the all-purpose rehabilitation centres is likely to fail from the start. The trouble is that of a good idea with inadequate research and what I believe to be a faulty answer. In fact, no-one can prove this either way as yet, which is why a rather more inquiring experimental approach might have been better. It seems to me quite possible that district hospital rehabilitation centres run the risk of being as poorly utilized, as the industrial rehabilitation centres often are.

Rehabilitation in its widest sense is truly an immensely important subject, and one which tends to be neglected. It requires a change in attitude of mind, away from interest in the acute episode, to encourage the patient to return to his or her former activities. It covers the period between recovery from disease and return to normal activities but, being of the nature of a 'follow-through', rehabilitation ought, I feel, to be retained in part as an interest of each involved specialty. Apart from difficulties in continuity of care, a separate rehabilitation specialty might also introduce an extra link in a sometimes difficult chain of communication. Many of the paramedical staff working in rehabilitation feel that doctors ordering treatment do not, in fact, understand what their particular activity in rehabilitation can offer to patients. There is a feeling that much of the treatment ordered is inappropriate whilst paramedical staff have considerable diffidence in advising doctors of what they feel would be the most appropriate lines of treatment. In fact, basic medical education involves little instruction in what the paramedical services involved in rehabilitation can offer and this would appear to me to be at the root of this communication difficulty.

I believe that rehabilitation is important in many different fields. Although through our lack of knowledge it has become a subject which we tend to ignore and to hope that someone else (often a geriatrician) will do for us, I believe that rehabilitation has an immense amount to offer in the fields of coronary thrombosis, cerebrovascular accident (so often managed sub-optimally), rheumatoid arthritis, and psychiatric illness, apart from physical trauma. I believe, however, that the needs of these interests differ in both kind and quantity. No-one would argue against the special needs for spinal injuries rehabilitation centres, and the same is true of each other type of disability which may benefit from rehabilitation.

Rehabilitation has not been a major field of medical interest, and I do not suggest that the present, irregular system of rehabilitation centres does not need considerable improvement in organization, facilities offered, and in the range of conditions treated. What I do fear is that the suggestion of regional or district rehabilitation centres may not only not work effectively, but may work to the detriment of the limited facilities which exist already. In other words, I believe that we should consider other ways of expanding our interest in this field. I believe that the proposed system is based on administrative convenience, rather than the needs of patients. Administratively, it is very tidy and, while agreeing that this is a virtue, I do not feel that it relates well to what is best for the patients the service is intended to serve.

The essence of medical rehabilitation is enthusiastic teamwork. This is a difficult atmosphere to create, and it will be even more difficult in specialties associated with prolonged disability than in acute trauma. The service has never yet been adequate even for acute trauma.

If rehabilitation is to become a specialty in its own right it implies that we must have medical specialists in rehabilitation. It seems that as in casualty their background will not be important; what will matter is their enthusiasm for rehabilitation, they must be able to work with their colleagues and with the many professions, ancillary to medicine which are involved in the rehabilitation field. This implies health care teams, it also implies case conferences where the problems of individual patients can be discussed between rehabilitation specialists, the specialist involved in the disorder from which the patient is being rehabilitated and the ancillary staff. Case conferences will have to discuss not only the physical aspect of rehabilitation but also the psychological and social aspect as well.

One major difficulty in the rehabilitation field is that the professions involved in rehabilitation are in disarray and have been largely ignored in the reorganization of the health service. A particular difficulty is that many of these careers have been regarded as suitable careers for young ladies, with financial rewards being of secondary importance. This is responsible for the poor financial state of these professions, now those who work in these groups have to work for their living, and find in common with other persons who work in National Health Services that they can no longer afford to subsidize the service. This is why these professions are in recruitment difficulties. Even when qualified, trained members of these professions find that they can no longer afford to work in the service; what they need, in fact, is a career structure. This implies that someone must be in command at regional level to work with the regional medical specialists in rehabilitation, subordinates will have to be in command at area level, and under them should come team leaders to be in charge of the differing sectors in the field of rehabilitation. Such an establishment would greatly facilitate training in the professions involved in rehabilitation which include physiotherapists, remedial gymnasts, speech therapists, social workers, clinical psychologists, and occupational therapists.

Each special field of rehabilitation requires a different mix of the above and perhaps in large centres several specialist fields of rehabilitation could be incorporated under the same roof. To me, however, this would appear to be of secondary importance; to me the important feature is the establishment of effective training and structure in the professions ancillary to medicine. As in casualty this is a field where health care is synonymous with teamwork.

The duty of the consultant in rehabilitation is to be in command of a team and to provide effective liaison (I have suggested case conferences might be necessary) with the consultants in the specialties involved. The difficulties both of the ancillary staff and of the medical staff, however, lie in the establishment of training schemes.

The last subject is the European Economic Community. Since this country joined the Community, we are now doctors working within the EEC. How our colleagues in Europe work, are treated, and act is therefore of great interest and importance to us. This is what being a member of a great profession is about. We stand or fall together. If one member fails, then we are all diminished in stature. If a member achieves greatness and honour, then this is reflected on the profession as a whole. No one of us can ignore safely the difficulties of a colleague in different circumstances from ourselves. I do not know where the Common Market will go, but I believe that the Common Market, Europe united, offers us our best chance of social and economic progress. The ideal of a united Europe is an old one and, for many hundreds of years, men of medicine travelled in Europe, maintaining the common

European heritage in our medical practice. This developed into a system of studies in which a doctor would visit centres such as Edinburgh, Vienna, and Padua in the course of furthering his medical education. I was encouraged in a surgical career by a translation of the diary of C. B. Tilanus (later to become professor of surgery in Amsterdam), who graduated from Utrecht in 1818. On graduating, he visited several clinics in Belgium, France, and Germany, observing and making notes on the activities of such men as Dupuytren, Langenbeck, and Marjolin. Many of the father figures of British medicine trained in the same way: a classical example is John Hunter. This pattern of postgraduate training was slowed down by the formation of the General Medical Council which in effect acted as a tariff barrier to freedom of movement in medical practice. Travel in Europe was further restricted by the First World War and stopped by the Second. We should, however, always remember the large numbers of medical refugees from Nazi-occupied Europe who have practised successfully in the United Kingdom, often with extreme distinction.

The three Articles of the Treaty of Rome which are of most interest to us are Article 57 (providing for the mutual recognition of diplomas), Article 48 (providing for the free migration of workers), and Article 63 (rendering it illegal to raise barriers to free migration). We tend to take a rather frightened, schizoid view of this. On the one hand, there is the opportunity of higher salaries and often better conditions of work should we migrate and, on the other hand, we fear that doctors who migrate here might not 'fit in'. The first vision is possible, as most doctors in other EEC countries earn vastly more than we do in this country. If this type of migration went on to any extent, our shortage specialities, such as radiology and anaesthetics, could be in great difficulty. It is probably true also that it would be most easy to migrate if one were practising in one of these fields, where subtleties of language are not quite so important and where British training is acknowledged to be supreme. The second vision is much less likely, as the earnings differential is too great. Last autumn, in Brussels, the British proposal for a committee to advise the commission on standards was accepted. This was a great advance on the six years or 5,500 hours allowed for basic medical education, which had been suggested in the draft directives previously.

The Permanent Committee of Doctors of the Common Market has two major sub-groups, UEMO (which covers the field of general practice) and UEMS (for specialist practitioners). UEMS also has mono-specialist sub-committees. The Permanent Committee is also concerned with the workings of the various health care systems as they affect the profession and the patient. Comprehensive health care systems exist, which are financed more directly by the consumer than our system of finance from the fund of general taxation. It is possible that some of these schemes are more efficient and, indeed, since they are not quite so limited by budgetary considerations, more comprehensive than our National Health Service. It is also possible that a greater awareness of the cost of health care by the consumer may tend to reduce frivolous demands of the service. We have the basis of a well-integrated health care system but it is grossly under-financed, as is shown by the relatively low proportion of the gross national product it receives.

Entry to the EEC does not guarantee free health care to visitors from Britain as yet, except in Denmark where we have a bilateral agreement. This is undoubtedly unfair, and efforts are being made to establish further bilateral agreements. This will take time.

The mutual recognition of basic medical qualifications should, theoretically, present few problems. No-one at international meetings ever states that a doctor is not a proper doctor because he qualified in a particular country. I feel that, with the advice which will be contained in the medical directives, this will present few problems. It has been suggested that there should be a period of adaptation which would enable a migrating doctor to become acquainted with the social manners and ethics of the recipient country. Since we cannot claim that the clinical attachment scheme has been a success, I would prefer the suggestion made by the British Medical Students' Association for information centres.

There has been a good deal of misunderstanding over the term 'specialist' in the United Kingdom. A specialist in European terms is a doctor who has completed an approved course of post-graduate training, varying in length according to specialty. Having undertaken this period of training, a doctor becomes 'a specialist': a protected title, giving the holder the right to charge higher fees and to have independent practice as a specialist. If, however, he wishes to look after patients in a public hospital, he has to become attached to a *chef de service*, or his equivalent. A *chef de service* is a little above the mean for seniority of the consultant grade. Thus, things are very different but, from the point of view of prospects for a specialist in training, the outlook is, on the whole, much better than in this country. A specialist migrating to this country soon after achieving his title may be expected to compete for registrar or senior registrar posts. On the other hand, if he had been an assistant for a suitable period, he would obviously be eligible to compete for consultant posts. As always, it would be more likely for a home candidate to obtain a post, but this could not be held to contravene Article 63. The reverse situation would apply to our nationals migrating elsewhere. This flow is much more likely, because of the great disparity in earnings. Our graduates would not get the best posts in the first instance, but they would obtain posts with much higher salaries attached than they could hope to achieve here. Even if they have never become *chef de service* they would be financially well off and would not suffer from the stigma which has been attached to any possible sub-consultant grade in this country.

A major difference between specialist practice in the United Kingdom and in Europe is that in most European countries patients have direct access to specialists and the GP need not be consulted first. Several of the EEC countries recognize general practice as a specialty, and UEMO has recommended two years' specialist training: it is this figure which is likely to appear in the directives. Thus, when the medical directives are established, a GP would be free to migrate as a GP after two years' specialist training. If, however, a recipient country had already established, as we are doing, three years' training, a migrant would have to fulfil the criteria of the recipient country; ie if migrating here, a further year's training would be required. Again, this is a highly theoretical problem, as very few will come. A doctor established before the ratification of the directives would have to demonstrate that he had carried out independent practice for twice the training period.

One of the great benefits of EEC entry is that it forces us to evaluate and compare our National Health Service with other health care systems. Even though medical practice differs throughout Europe, we do share the same philosophy, and we must actively further the interest of a European medical profession.

This would be helped by exchanges of pre- and postgraduate students, and by exchanges of established doctors. I look forward to the day when the 'been to Utrecht' comes to be regarded as having the same value as the 'been to America' has today. We must stand together in a united European profession. If any one of us feels that the standards or conditions of work of another doctor in another field in another area or country are not our concern, then we are laying the profession open to manipulation by governments. This will not only have an adverse effect upon every one of us, but also upon each patient who, from time to time, comes under our care.

In terms of 1969 figures I would hope that the following statistical information which is taken from *Health Care: The Growing Dilemma*, a report by Robert Maxwell working on behalf of McKinsey, would help to enable readers to compare the position of the United Kingdom in the health care league.

National cost in US $ per head of population

United Kingdom	93
England and Wales	—
Italy	81
Republic of Ireland	77
Netherlands	116
France	150
West Germany	154
Sweden	234
United States	298

In percentage of gross national product

United Kingdom	4·6
England and Wales	—
Italy	5·2
Republic of Ireland	—
Netherlands	5·9
France	5·7
West Germany	5·7
Sweden	6·4
United States	6·7

Numbers of doctors per 10,000 population

United Kingdom	—
England and Wales	12·3
Italy	18·1
Republic of Ireland	—
Netherlands	12·5
France	13·2
West Germany	17·2
Sweden	13·6
United States	15·8

Hospital beds per 10,000 population

United Kingdom	—
England and Wales	95
Italy	105
Republic of Ireland	128
Netherlands	97
France	100
West Germany	111
Sweden	164
United States	81

Average length of stay in hospital in days

England and Wales	11·1
Italy	13·4
Netherlands	17·9
France	18·0
West Germany	18·5

Sweden	12·6
United States	9·3

Average bed occupancy (%)	
England and Wales	79
Italy	77
Netherlands	94·2
France	77·9
West Germany	86·9
Sweden	75·7
United States	74·9

Percentage cost of health care provided as personal expenditure or personal insurance cover	
United Kingdom	7
Italy	78
France	33
Netherlands	34·6
West Germany	26·9
Sweden	7
United States	64·6

To compare population of those countries per square kilometre	
England and Wales	303
Republic of Ireland	40
Netherlands	342
France	83
Italy	164
West Germany	215
Sweden	17
United States	19

Infant mortality per 1,000 live-births	
England and Wales	23·7
Republic of Ireland	26·1
Netherlands	19·6
France	25·4
Italy	32·4
West Germany	25·2
Sweden	16·3
United States	27·1

Maternal mortality per 100,000 live-births	
England and Wales	19·4
Netherlands	19·4
France	24·9
Italy	60·6
West Germany	53·1
Republic of Ireland	31·8
Sweden	10·2
United States	24·5

Finally, I must return to my original topic and observe that organizations such as the Nuffield Provincial Hospitals Trust exist to attempt to make progress where the NHS, with its restricting budgeting, cannot risk money. Many people in the NHS have excellent ideas for its improvement. Ideas may originate from administration or from the profession; the ideas of an administrator can be put into practice only if the profession can be persuaded to accept them. This leads the administrator into the twin temptations of selecting the members of the advisory committees, or giving the profession inadequate time to discuss lengthy documents. On the other hand, good ideas arising from the profession, if not in line with departmental policy, are unlikely to gain acceptance. The purpose of the

Nuffield Provincial Hospitals Trust is to smooth over these difficulties and to allow for experiment, without which there can be no progress. Without such an organization, I believe that the NHS would be so rigid that it would become unworkable. It provides one of the few flexible areas for medical practice in this country, and I must thank them for allowing me so free a hand to write on how I see various aspects of the prognosis of health care in this country.

A further feature of this aspect of health care systems is that even vast sums of money and manpower spent on health care do not guarantee a uniformly good service; indeed it can be argued that the reverse is the case. Wealthy areas became centres of excellence which attracted even more funds and manpower than they already started with. This is undoubtedly to the detriment of other areas. It is in fact impossible to demonstrate objectively that the NHS has had any significant impact on the nation's health or that it is good value for money.

In the preparation of this essay I must gratefully acknowledge that I have received much help and advice from a wide variety of friends and colleagues working in many fields of health care. In particular I should like to acknowledge advice received from Mr Cyril Slack, orthopaedic surgeon in charge, Hartford Hall, Miners' Rehabilitation Centre; Dr E. Woodford Williams, director, National Health Service, Hospital Advisory Service; Sir George Godber, Mr Gordon MacLachlan of the Nuffield Provincial Hospitals Trust; and Dr Ian Mckim Thompson, Regional Secretary, British Medical Association, Birmingham Regional Office.

REFERENCES

MAXWELL, ROBERT (1974). *Health Care: The Growing Dilemma* (New York: McKinsey & Co.).

WILLIAMS, E. WOODFORD (1972). 'Rehabilitation: the problem in the old', *Proc. R. Soc. Med.* 65.

Community medicine

DULCIE GOODING

DULCIE GOODING
MB, BS, MFCM, DPH
Area Medical Officer

Community medicine

The history of medicine during the last century has seen the evolution of a wide range of specialties. To give but a few examples, widely differing specialties such as paediatrics and geriatrics have developed from general medicine and gynaecology from surgery. By a similar process of evolution the new specialty of community medicine has developed over the past six years.

Community medicine is concerned with 'the application of medicine to whole populations or to defined groups and hence with the ascertainment of health needs and how professional services can best be organized to meet these needs'. This concept was clearly enunciated by the Royal Commission on Medical Education in 1968 (1), at a time when the future of public health, social medicine, and medical administration, the precursors of community medicine, were under close scrutiny. There are many countries where the full-time involvement of doctors in the management and development of health services has virtually ceased or remains only on a small and ineffective scale. In this country, by 1968, for reasons which will be described, the future of such activities was uncertain. Some of the components of the specialty had existed under a variety of guises, depending on the orientation and responsibilities of the practitioners concerned. Recruitment to these was unsatisfactory, largely on account of the inadequate definition of roles, inappropriate training, and poor career prospects, particularly in the public health service. The last six years, however, have seen a substantial change, and today the specialty is at last ready to attain full recognition as a distinct discipline within the broad field of medicine. With the reorganization of the NHS the specialty in its new form has much to contribute and has great opportunities for development and for attaining its wide potential.

The first concepts relevant to community medicine developed in the early Victorian era. The Industrial Revolution resulted in the depopulation of agricultural areas and in the rapid unplanned growth of the big cities: London doubled in size from just under one million to two million people between 1801 and 1841. These developments were accompanied by problems of malnutrition, continuing epidemics of infectious disease, and a multiplicity of social evils. The review of environmental and social conditions undertaken in the early part of the century by Chadwick led to the appointment of Dr W. Duncan in Liverpool and Dr (later Sir John) Simon in the City of London in 1847 and 1848, respectively, as the first medical officers of health; within ten years nearly all local government districts had made similar appointments.

At central government level a General Board of Health was established, which was eventually succeeded by a medical department of the Privy Council. These central organizations influenced public health work in the periphery in many directions, including the distribution of general guidance, in much the same way as the DHSS provides help and advice to those in the field today. For example, the original advice on the duties of medical officers of health was drawn up in consultation with doctors just as consultation between the central government and the medical profession takes place nowadays. Another pattern of development in health services also emerged, still common today, whereby major extensions of policy and activity were often administrative in conception and accomplishment, whereas major advances in curative medicine continued to come from individual clinicians.

Great progress was made and no community physician of the future will have the satisfaction of seeing the mortality statistics fall so dramatically largely as a result of his labours; the rewards in future will be far more difficult to measure and more subtle in nature. The medical officer of health of the past was dependent to a substantial degree, as is the community physician today, on others to provide him with essential information on the incidence of disease. As early as the mid 1600s Graunt, a member of the Royal Society, a draper by trade, analysed Bills of Mortality and for the first time drew conclusions from statistical data. In the 1800s, epidemiological studies were undertaken by Snow, Simon, and William Farr, the last-named being the first medical statistician to the Registrar General's office; their reports on the incidence and causes of disease were utilized by a Royal Commission whose report resulted in the Public Health Acts of 1866, 1872, and 1875; much of this legislation relating to the control of the environment was incorporated into the Public Health Act of 1936, a substantial part of which is still in use.

On the hospital side, religious orders had established hospitals in the Middle Ages and by the nineteenth century many hospitals, including most of the teaching hospitals, were run by voluntary, religious, or charitable organizations. In parallel with these developments the State, by the nineteenth century, was establishing general and infectious disease hospitals and, more particularly, mental illness and mental subnormality institutions through boards of guardians. On the administrative side, medical superintendents were appointed to these hospitals and became involved in their planning and organization but, unlike medical officers of health, had little or nothing to do with the development of preventive services. The hospitals run by the boards of guardians were taken over by the local authorities after 1929 but the separate municipal and voluntary components of the hospital service were not unified until the establishment of the NHS in 1948. Then, with the exception of psychiatric and a few large general hospitals, medical superintendent posts began to lapse in England and Wales, although many were retained in Scotland, leaving something of a gap on the medical administrative side within the English hospital system until the medical executive committee structure began to develop with increasing rationality in the 1960s.

By the beginning of the twentieth century the immediate and pressing problems of the control of infectious disease and the improvement of the environment were beginning to diminish. The medical officer of health had a public health inspectorate working with him on the environmental side. Social reformers such as Shaftesbury and Booth had already set the trends for the development of many of the personal health and social services. In 1902, the Midwives Act gave responsibility to local health authorities for the registration and supervision of midwives. Child health facilities were developing, at first as a result of voluntary effort and later as part of the local authority health services. The district nursing service was established in the late 1800s and the health visiting service in the first decade of the new century, although these services were fragmentary in the early stages of development, relying heavily on local and voluntary support. In 1907, the school medical service was established following a report on the poor condition of potential recruits for the Boer War; this service made provision, *inter alia*, for the ascertainment of handicapped children and for the provision of certain minor treatment facilities. School health services, modified to meet the very changed needs, still function today by virtue of their inclusion in the 1944 and subsequent Education Acts. Other recommendations included in this survey and implemented in following years related to school meals, regulation of conditions of work for women and children, provision of maternity benefits and registration of still-births.

In 1907, notification of births was made statutory, a service on which the medical officer of health depended to ensure that supervision and care were made promptly available to children and mothers in need, and which he has also utilized in more recent years to set up computerized immunization systems and serial developmental assessments at child health clinics. These and other services were the responsibility of the medical officer of health and, in this period, his involvement in the planning, organization, and day-to-day management of both preventive and curative services was extensive. He was the executive officer responsible for the measures undertaken to control outbreaks of infectious disease; he was the person responsible for determining the clinical work to be undertaken in the school health and child health services; and, together with his medical and nursing colleagues, he was deeply involved in the evolution of the day-to-day clinical work undertaken by all community nursing staff, including midwives in the days when the majority of deliveries still took place at home, although in many instances community nursing staff were employed by the voluntary associations up until 1948.

In 1911, Lloyd George's Insurance Act entitled contributors to sickness benefit and to GP services, the latter being inopportunely commemorated by the design of the medical record envelopes still in use in general practice. Provision was also made for developing chest clinics and building sanatoria for those suffering from tuberculosis, and services were developed for the control of venereal disease. The work of the medical officer of health therefore continued to expand and his hospital involvement was extensive from 1929 until 1948. As growing numbers of services were created and expanded, the medical officer of health also became responsible, on behalf of the local health authority, for the employment of staff from many different professional disciplines, including paramedical staff and sometimes social workers.

In 1919, the Ministry of Health was established and, from then until 1939, that Ministry was heavily committed in the field of environmental health and the control of infectious disease. It was also, however, increasingly involved in the maternity and child health service and in the hospital service, including cancer programmes; and links were being forged in the international field. From 1938 the central department became concerned with the provision of emergency hospitals and with the need for developing countrywide provision for medical care in time of war. As a result of this the Ministry became involved in the recruitment of doctors interested in the organization and planning of health care, no longer drawing almost solely from the ranks of the Public Health Service as in earlier years.

Following the Beveridge Report in 1943 and a working group to consider a national health service in 1944, the country and, after initial protestations, the majority of the medical profession were ready to accept an organized national health service, which came into being in 1948. In the early years of the Service, at central level, the Ministry of Health was preoccupied with the development of hospitals and specialist services; the GP services, having jealously guarded their independent contractor status in 1948, remained relatively uninvolved at this stage in the over-all development of the health service. The local authorities also maintained relative independence from the central department, although development schemes were often submitted for approval, especially when financial loans were required.

The setting up of the NHS coincided with the start of another period of rapid scientific and technical advance, together with the availability of a growing range of curative drugs. These developments played their part in encouraging the evolution of subspecialties within general medicine and surgery and helped to maintain the gulf which existed between different branches of the service, which was perpetuated by the new tripartite structure. It must be borne in mind, however, that the tripartite structure had pulled together a highly fragmented service. On the hospital side, however, new posts were created at regional level for administrative medical officers. In the first decade of the NHS, the regional hospital boards were heavily committed in the development of specialist services and the number of consultants increased steadily with a more equitable distribution of specialties throughout the country. By the 1960s the boards were getting absorbed in the physical planning and building of hospitals; and it is only in recent years that the medical staff at regional level have taken an increasing interest in service planning, although the degree of commitment has varied throughout the country. By the 1960s the regional hospital board medical officers were active in the development of postgraduate medical training programmes, working in close liaison with the postgraduate deans of their universities. They were also involved, probably with less success, in the development of training for paramedical staff.

Local health authority boundaries remained unaltered in 1948, and varied considerably in population from some 30,000 to over two million. It is not surprising therefore that the work undertaken by medical officers of health likewise varied throughout the country. In 1948, the medical officers of health lost their direct involvement with the hospital service, their remaining links being in many instances only as members of hospital management committees.

In the following twenty-five years, local authority health departments had to adapt to further changes, modifying and withdrawing some services and developing others. Efficient immunization programmes, together with the use of potent drugs, reduced the load of infectious disease on both community and hospital services; tuberculosis is perhaps the best example. Continual retraining of existing staff and recruitment of staff from professions new to the community service have been part of the pattern. The public health inspectorate worked increasingly as an independent profession, looking to the medical officer of health only for medical advice; under reorganization they remain as employees of local government. The community nursing staff, particularly following the implementation of the Mayston Report, gradually developed their own management structure and have accepted responsibility for the training, deployment, and standards of clinical care of their own staff. The growing specialty of social work attained professional independence with the implementation of the Seebohm Report and the creation of the new social service departments throughout the country in 1970. In many instances this last change involved the division of joint health and welfare departments which had been the responsibility of the medical officer of health. The continual fragmentation of the local authority health departments was understandably stressful for the staff concerned, and recruitment to the service began to fall a decade or more ago.

Paradoxically, during the same period a growing number of enlightened medical officers of health came to realize that they could utilize the flexibility of policy which in turn stemmed from flexibility in finance, inherent in their being employees of local government. In particular they began to bring their services into closer relationship with general practice on the one hand and with the hospital service on the other, thereby achieving a more integrated and hence better standard of care for patients (2, 3).

On the GP side, a major contribution towards this process lay in schemes of attachment of nursing teams, containing a range of professional skills, to practices. Before this, health visitors, nurses, and midwives employed by local health authorities had looked after geographical areas, with the result that one nurse might have to provide care for the patients of a dozen or more GPs; and by the same token, a single practitioner might find that patients in different parts of his practice were receiving the attention of a similar number of nurses (4). By making possible schemes of attachment, medical officers of health facilitated a team approach to the care of patients in the community. Within such teams it became possible to re-define roles, with the result that nurses had the opportunity for accepting wider responsibilities, with consequential increased job satisfaction, whilst at the same time helping to ensure that the doctors' specific skills were used to best effect.

The second field in which medical officers of health have assisted the evolution of general practice has been through the health centre building programme. In 1948, it had been envisaged by many of the proponents of the NHS that primary care would come to be delivered from health centres rather than from the traditional doctors' surgeries. For a variety of reasons this change did not begin on an appreciable scale for fifteen years. Since then, however, there has been a steadily rising demand for health centres from GPs and it has been the task of the medical officer of health to arrange for their provision. The significance of health centres lies not in a rehousing of doctors into resplendent new premises in which they simply continue to practise in a time-honoured fashion, but rather in the opportunities they offer for the establishment of well-organized primary care teams.

On the hospital side, many medical officers of health have likewise been active. Schemes for the planned early discharge of certain surgical patients and for a conjoint system of hospital and community obstetric care have been developed. In psychiatry and in the growing problem of geriatric care, public health doctors have likewise been involved with their hospital colleagues and, of course, with GPs in the development of systems of continuing care in the hospital and community. In diseases which call for surveillance and the education of patients, such as diabetes mellitus, systems of care and after-care by specially trained health visitors have been developed at the instigation of or in co-operation with medical officers of health.

In addition to his integrative role, the medical officer of health has, of course, had to maintain and develop services for which he and his staff were responsible and which were not yet ripe for integration with clinical medicine either at primary care or hospital level. The notable examples are the child and school health services and a substantial amount of pioneering work has been undertaken in the field of developmental paediatrics and in the evolution of multidisciplinary team assessment of the handicapped. Other services which have been developed by medical officers of health have included health education programmes and family planning services.

The main contribution, however, has lain in the gradual pulling together of what had previously been the three functional disparate branches of the NHS; likewise doctors employed on the administrative side of the hospital service have come to realize that it is illogical and often fruitless to confine the application of their administrative skills to a single segment of the NHS in isolation from the other two. The more general appreciation of this fact is indeed one of the factors which underlies the recent reorganization of the service.

COMMUNITY MEDICINE IN THE REORGANIZED HEALTH SERVICE

By 1968, the twentieth anniversary of the inauguration of the NHS, functional integration of the three branches was well under way and administrative unification was under active discussion. Late that year the government published the first Green Paper (5), a rather unusual form of publication, since repeated in other fields, which allowed for consultation and discussion with interested public and professional organizations prior to making final recommendations. This advocated the establishment of area boards throughout the country, 40 to 50 in number, ranging from three-quarters of a million to two or three million population in size. It considered that these area authorities should be responsible for the total health services in the areas which they served. The area authorities were to be sufficiently removed from day-to-day operations 'to take a wide view of the need for efficiency in their service and the requirements of the service'. The area boards would include community medicine specialists with particular responsibilities for the planning and operation of services. A district level was to be created to manage the service on a day-to-day basis. The idea of the single tier of authority which allowed for easy flow from the then Ministry of Health to the area health boards was attractive to many prospective community physicians and many considered the proposed population size of the areas a realistic one in which to work.

In 1970, a second Green Paper (6) was published. This concluded that there should be 90 area health authorities and that there was need for a further planning level at region; 14 regional health councils would therefore be responsible for the over-all planning and allocation of major resources and also for co-ordination of postgraduate medical education and training. As in the previous paper, it was recommended that the day-to-day organization and management of the service should be delegated to a district level. It emphasized for the first time the importance of relating the area level of organization to that of reorganized local government.

The following year a Consultative Document (7) was published and gave particular emphasis to the need for an effective management structure within the health service, in order to make the best use of scarce resources both of money and of manpower. The Consultative Document also acknowledged the special needs of teaching districts, and allowed for the continuation of many of the functions of local executive councils in the guise of family practitioner committees to deal with the pay and conditions of service of GPs outside the mainstream of health service management. It proposed the development, at district level, of community health councils to strengthen public participation which in the NHS, with the exception of local health authorities, has in the past always been weak.

Potential community medicine specialists watched the emerging proposals for health service reorganization with keen interest. It was clear that there would be a new role for them under reorganization and they held positive, if varying, views of the administrative suggestions. The medical profession questioned the role of the clinician in management, as well as the role of the community medicine specialist in relation to the development of clinical services, both preventive and curative. There was also argument about the level at which the various management and planning roles of the new service could best be fulfilled. The debate continued and, understandably, future community medicine specialists in the field felt frustrated and insecure.

Publication of the Hunter Report (8) in 1972 helped to clarify some of the problems. This report picked out five key areas of knowledge required by community medicine specialists of the future: namely medicine and human biology; epidemiology and environmental health; statistics; social and behavioural sciences; social administration; and health service management.

The role in management has always been contentious because clinicians, and especially GPs, are quite correctly wary of losing clinical autonomy. Recognizing, however, quite clearly the size, cost, and complexity of the health service, the Hunter Working Party specifically stated that involvement in management was a key part of the community medicine specialist's responsibilities, whilst clinical responsibility was a matter exclusively for the practitioner.

Publication of the Grey Book on management (9) in late 1972 did something to clarify these problems, although as is inevitable in any major reorganization, many compromises had been reached. This Grey Book made the most indigestible reading but at least began to spell out in some detail the role of the various professional staff after reorganization. On the management side it described for the first time the consensus decision-making role of the new teams of officers at the various levels, the doctor, nurse, treasurer, and administrator forming a team. This is a new concept in the health service and time will tell whether it improves the quality and efficiency of decision-making. There are so many possibilities; in some teams personalities will dominate either constructively or destructively, although in the district management teams where three doctors are present (a community medicine specialist, a GP, and consultant) it would be reasonable to assume that the medical view might predominate.

In general the concept of consensus team working has been accepted, and a remarkable degree of goodwill exists to make the new management structure work. It is only in times of a major clinical emergency, such as a smallpox outbreak, that it would be imperative that the doctor should, on a temporary basis, lead the team. The non-hierarchal structure of the new specialty of community medicine also emerged during reorganization. Previously, for example, the medical officer of health was always directly accountable for all his staff, medical, paramedical, nursing, and administrative. The new organization will relate more to the old regional hospital board structure where the senior administrative medical officer was regarded by his clinical, administrative, and nursing colleagues as a co-equal. This type of organization can, of course, have its frustrations. Decision-making could, in an unhappy team, become very difficult and the area health authority would have a problem on its hands. Intelligently used, however, there need be no difficulties and policy recommendations should benefit from the balanced consideration of the team.

The White Paper and the Bill for reorganization of the health service were published in rapid succession, in late 1972, and reorganization on 1 April 1974, became a reality. In the early stages of the reorganized health service, community medicine specialists will be required to fill a variety of posts.

At regional level, a specialist will be needed in health service planning, with particular emphasis on project work related to the development and building of hospitals; a second specialist with a particular interest in service planning; a third skilled in information systems and research techniques; and a fourth interested in medical staffing, manpower, and training, and also postgraduate medical education.

At area level, posts will be available for specialists skilled in the development of child health services; the development, in liaison with local authority social service departments, of adult health services, which include care of the elderly and the mentally and physically handicapped; and a third specialist skilled in service planning and information systems.

At both regional and area levels senior medical staff will be appointed, whose prime responsibility will be to co-ordinate the work of these specialists, although as in other fields of medicine, the regional medical officer and area medical officer will not be directly accountable for the specialist work of their community medicine colleagues.

At district level, a district community physician will be appointed to participate in the day-to-day management of the service, and to help in establishing the health care planning teams responsible for initiating planning proposals. He will also be responsible to the local authority for the environmental health of the community, including the former medical officer of health's role in the control of infectious disease.

The number of consultant posts to be established in England and Wales in the early years of reorganization is therefore limited, and as with consultant posts in the clinical field, the number and type will ultimately be controlled at central level, by machinery negotiated between the profession and the DHSS. It must be noted, however, that, owing to poor recruitment in the past to the forerunners of community medicine, it may be difficult to fill all the initial specialist posts, bearing in mind the need to achieve and maintain satisfactory standards.

Some indication of the possible scale of development is given in the Scottish Home and Health Department's publication *Community Medicine in Scotland* (10) where the working group saw the need for up to sixteen specialists in community medicine for an area of 400,000 population with two districts. The Scottish report recommends the division of community medicine specialists in such an area into three parts: one concerned with planning and management of services; a second with special commitments such as information services, environmental health and health education; and a third comprising two district teams, each of three specialists. It must be borne in mind that Scotland, under reorganization, has no regional tier but, even so, it is doubtful if in England and Wales sufficient skills would be available to fill an analogous number of posts at specialist level in the immediate future. In terms of manpower planning it is also to be hoped that community medicine will not get into the same difficulties as other branches of medicine in the past by creating an excessive number of junior staff in relation to consultant posts.

In England and Wales, having regard to the decline of experience in the epidemiology and control of communicable disease, it may well prove desirable to introduce at regional level, and possibly in conjunction with the Public Health Laboratory Service, a source of skilled advice which would be available when required for community medicine specialists with district responsibilities. There are also the more esoteric aspects of environmental health in which expertise is even scarcer, being currently largely concentrated at central level and in a limited number of universities and research institutions. Here again, it is desirable to plan for the availability of expert help at regional or more likely at supra-regional level. A third and vital group of skills relates to information systems and here a regional grouping seems logical, at least in the first instance. Whilst the gathering and utilization of data would be of major importance at area level, processing and interpretation call for facilities and expert knowledge, which it would be wasteful to deploy below regional level. A highly skilled team, which should include an epidemiologist, a medical statistician, and computer programmers, with a grasp of health service organizational problems, should be recruited to regional level. Formal links should be created between this regional team and the community medicine specialist at area level responsible for the planning and development of information systems. These teams should also be responsible for the development, with their clinical colleagues, of modern record and filing systems for use both in general practice and hospital work. For epidemiological use and planning purposes the data collected must be in comparable form.

THE PRACTICALITIES OF COMMUNITY MEDICINE

Having described the formal proposals for fitting community medicine into the administrative structure of the reorganized

NHS, it might be useful to try to group the functions of community physicians under three broad headings and then to recount some personal experiences in a situation akin to that of such a specialist.

Whilst there have been numerous publications (11, 12, 13) discussing the potential functions of a community physician, the latter can conveniently be classified under the headings of epidemiology, interpretation, and innovation. Epidemiology is the basic discipline on which depends the assessment of health within a community or in special groups of the population and the measurement of the effects on them of environmental and other influences, including the nature and quality of local health services. By his training in the epidemiological approach, the community physician should be able to assist his clinical and other colleagues to assess the problems with which they are faced and to ascertain the outcome of attempts to solve or to relieve them.

The interpretive role has several facets. It is, for example, necessary, again as part of a team, to try to predict the consequences of advances in medical knowledge, as these often have substantial implications for resources, both of skilled manpower and of buildings and equipment. For example, the advent of intermittent haemodialysis has had a substantial effect on resources both within the hospital and in the domiciliary setting. Similarly, the result of neonatal surgery in spina bifida has produced long-term consequences, not merely in relation to health services, but also to social work and educational services. It will be the task of the community physician to assist in interpreting the likely consequences of such advances and to help in planning to cope with them. There will also be an important interpretive role to play between the health services on the one hand, and the local authority social and educational services on the other, in relation to such groups as the physically and mentally handicapped or those in need of special educational treatment. Likewise there are important functions to be fulfilled in helping to relate the consequences of general social changes to health service requirements; as well as the consequences of health service developments for the community at large.

Innovation is certainly not the prerogative of the community physician, or for that matter of the doctor. Nevertheless, within medicine it is important that there should be some with special responsibilities towards studying contemporary systems of care with a view to ensuring that they are still as fully relevant as possible to needs. Should they fail to pass this test, alternative approaches would require to be considered and here again the community physician, with his particular background and skills, should be able to help his health service colleagues.

In all this the community physician should be seen not in any way as a competitor with clinicians, or with members of other professions, but rather as one whose skills will facilitate their work. In this connection it might be of interest to draw on personal experience acquired during five years spent in a post in many ways analogous to that of a community physician.

In 1967, it was decided that the new city of Milton Keynes should be established in north Buckinghamshire, involving the growth of population in the area from some 40,000 to 250,000 before the end of the century. The area in question had the usual range of primary care services, together with limited specialist out-patient facilities, and it was clear that there were both the opportunity and the need to develop a comprehensive health service on a district scale. There was general goodwill towards this suggestion, but a focus for health care planning was clearly necessary and this was established through a joint planning structure representing all three branches of the then tripartite NHS (14, 15). It was in turn necessary to provide this structure with a small administrative nucleus, the medical component of which comprised a post which, although formally within the public health service, also had links with the regional hospital board and GP services.

As the incumbent of this post, I found myself fulfilling a role analogous in many respects to that of the future community physician. The medical practitioners and others providing clinical services within the designated area of the proposed new town were interested in the suggested planning of a comprehensive health service for Milton Keynes, but readily accepted that they required the complementary help of a colleague whose experience included medical aspects of administration. It would have been understandable if some had been suspicious lest they should find their ways of working subjected to change, but such a reaction was rarely encountered, and an important aspect of the job was to convey the clear message that whatever plan might emerge was to be the result of a consensus. Happily, work was able to proceed successfully on that basis throughout the entire planning process.

The initial group concerned with planning included not only doctors but representatives of other health service professions, and a major task of the prototype community physician lay in encouraging and helping them to outline a broad philosophy of health care for the new city: whilst at the same time ensuring that they did not become lost in a welter of detail. The result of this joint endeavour was *A Health Service for Milton Keynes* (16) which was subsequently endorsed by all three statutory NHS bodies as the basis for the detailed planning which was to follow.

The community physician's next role lay in helping to establish a framework within which detailed plans for individual services could be worked out, and this involved the establishment of what are now known as health care planning teams. As these got under way it was necessary to provide them with a wide range of background information about the local situation but, in addition, regard had to be paid to developments elsewhere which might prove useful and relevant in the Milton Keynes situation. This latter activity could sometimes be achieved by the provision of reprints of relevant articles or by the production of a summary paper, but it also involved, on occasion, inviting experts from other parts of the country to contribute their experience to planning meetings.

It was important to keep in close touch with all that was happening through attendance at meetings of the health care planning teams in order to provide help and advice where required, and also to ensure that the detailed policies which were being formulated by the various teams were compatible with each other as well as with the over-all health service plan for the new city.

In addition to this planning work it was often found necessary to undertake individual discussions with clinical colleagues. For example, on the general practice side, many hours were spent discussing with family doctors and other members of the primary care team the numerous matters involved in the reorganization and development of the team in preparation for transfer to a health centre. Similar discussions with consultants took place, for example, on the balance of care in their respective specialties between the hospital and the health centre setting. On a wider front, it was also important to fulfil a liaison role between the health services on the one hand and, on the other, such agencies as social services, education departments, and those responsible for the over-all planning of the new city and its services, including housing, transport, and industry. A health service planned in isolation from the other social institutions of society would have been doomed to failure.

A particularly vital role lay in acting as one of the main links between the health service and members of the public. The latter were, of course, involved in membership of the statutory NHS authorities and a continuing dialogue was initiated to ensure that there was a full and mutual understanding of each other's points of view. On a wider scale there was the problem of keeping members of the local public in the picture and this involved participation in many meetings held in the existing towns, villages, and hamlets of the designated area. In the course of these, it was often found that there were fundamental misunderstandings of the aims and objectives of health services and also of what was practicable in terms of manpower and money. This task of interpreting medicine to the public will be of great importance in the work of community physicians throughout the country and the advent of community health councils should provide a stimulus to such work. There was, of course, a substantial input into many of these activities from those whose background was other than medical, but there is no doubt that there was regular scope for contributions from the specific point of view of community medicine.

ACADEMIC COMMUNITY MEDICINE

In addition to the divisions between different branches of the health service, which continued with the structuring of the tripartite service in 1948, there also developed an unfortunate schism between the applied and academic branches of public health. Before that time, instruction for medical students had largely been in the hands of medical officers of health, some of whom occupied part-time professorial chairs. As such posts on the academic side became vacant they were not uncommonly filled from the ranks of those whose interests were wider than those of medical officers of health of the time, and university departments increasingly assumed the title of social medicine rather than public health. The result was that those practising public health in the field became more and more devoid of academic stimulus and one evidence of this lay in their small output of research, without which any subject is liable to wither. University teachers of social medicine, on the other hand, unlike their clinical colleagues, often lacked experience in the practicalities of the subject which they taught; and attempts to remedy this by inviting certain medical officers of health to participate in teaching did not entirely resolve the problem.

One of the most encouraging of recent trends has been the increasing coming together of the academic and applied components of what is now community medicine. This has been accompanied by the direct involvement of certain university departments, not only in health service research but also in the provision, for example, of information and intelligence systems for some of the new health authorities. As the requisite skills in this field are scarce and largely concentrated in academic departments, such joint approaches will be of great benefit to the NHS, whilst at the same time providing for the access of such departments to suitable material both for teaching and for research. A temporary snag is that many academic units of community medicine are currently under-staffed; but, nevertheless, this is no argument against the development of joint appointments between them and service authorities.

UNDERGRADUATE TRAINING

During the past twenty years training of undergraduates in social medicine has left much to be desired in many medical schools. In the late 1950s the University of London, which trained almost 50 per cent of doctors in Great Britain, removed public health as a compulsory subject from the curriculum. The fact that only a minority of London medical schools have reinstated the related subject of social medicine to any real extent by establishing academic units does little to encourage an understanding of the specialty by the average undergraduate. The University, in fact, spends a quite substantial sum on research and training in community medicine at the London School of Hygiene but this has concentrated all the money and expertise on the postgraduate student. Medical schools in the rest of the country, fortunately, have a better record, as both undergraduate and postgraduate training take place together.

Added to this practical difficulty is the problem of evolving methods of teaching community medicine to undergraduates so that it is both comprehensible and interesting. The appeal of acute medicine and the care of individual patients are understandably more attractive to most young doctors. The community at large also thinks of medicine in these terms and is largely unaware of, or uninterested in, epidemiology, in the relationship between social problems and disease, in the heavy and increasing case-load of long-term care in the psychiatric and geriatric fields; and it is apathetic about many aspects of prevention. Young people are therefore often attracted to medicine with little or no understanding either of the fact that there are unmet needs or of where the heavy workload really lies. Similarly, they are unaware of the size and complexity of the health service and of the administrative machinery needed to enable it to fulfil its function. The health service is big business, and one of the largest employers of staff in the country, currently costing some £3,000 million per annum. Quite correctly medical students enter medicine intending to work with individual patients. It is important, however, that they learn during their training about their roles and responsibilities in the over-all situation, for the right and necessary clinical independence of every doctor should be accompanied, as described in the latest Cogwheel Report (17), by an understanding of the effects of his clinical decisions, in management terms, on the whole NHS.

In recent years the more progressive departments of social or community medicine have been looking at the problem of how best to teach their subject. The consensus of opinion is that the basic principles of epidemiology and statistics, together with sociology and psychology, should be taught in the early years. The teaching can take place either as a continuous process throughout pre-clinical training or as a series of short courses. The modern curricula in medicine at Southampton and Nottingham Universities include an introduction to some of the skills required to practise community medicine in the early years of training. For example, a study of carcinoma of the lung may include seminars in which a physician, a surgeon, and a pathologist, and also an epidemiologist and a health educator, can participate.

Some understanding of management and of the doctor's role within the health team is also desirable and practical experience in these latter fields might be acquired during the first two clinical years by attachment to, say, the district management team and their colleagues for a short period, and similar experience might also be gained at area and regional levels. It is, however, probably wise to bow to tradition and allow the student to concentrate on the study of clinical medicine during his final year.

A particularly hopeful sign for the future is the increasing social awareness of medical students; a knowledge of community medicine and also general practice, another sorely neglected subject in some medical schools, is easier to teach to students who are prepared to look at the position of the health service in relation to the over-all needs of society, rather than as a separate entity divorced from all else.

SPECIALIST POSTGRADUATE TRAINING

There are no basic differences in the skills employed in community medicine within the district, area, and regional tiers of the health service and in the DHSS. The Royal Commission on Medical Education recommended that entrants to the specialty should be well versed in clinical medicine and have had opportunities to study social factors in disease both within the hospital and in the general practice setting prior to entering the specialty. They also noted that experience in other subjects in some depth, particularly mentioning paediatrics and psychiatry, would contribute a useful background to further specialist training. Essentially similar conclusions were reached by the Hunter Committee. Community medicine already offers scope for particular interests which allow for the recruitment of a wide range of doctors with differing clinical backgrounds and personal leanings. It is quite acceptable that someone who is interested in, say, child health or care of the elderly may not have a bent towards developing the skills needed to improve medical recording, collection of statistics or utilization of computers. While a basic knowledge of those latter skills is required by every community physician, an in-depth grasp of the subject can be expected from only a proportion.

The Faculty of Community Medicine of the Royal Colleges of Physicians was established in 1972 and published an outline of their possible training requirements in 1973 (18). These followed the example of the parent colleges in that they envisaged the acquisition of Part I of the Membership as a foundation for higher specialist training and common to individuals practising community medicine who will include those working in health service administration, epidemiology, research, medical information systems, preventive medicine, environmental medicine, health education, or combinations of these subjects. There will also be specialists working in the community medicine aspects of child health and adult health, the latter with particular reference to the community care of the physically and mentally handicapped.

The Faculty envisage the academic training being acquired in a variety of different ways. One method would be through participation in a full-time course, an example of this being the MSc course at the London School of Hygiene. Another would be to undertake a series of planned appointments in the community medicine field, interspersed either with attendance at a part-time course or attending a series of academic modules and accompanied by supervised academic work. This last method has already been recognized by the setting up of modular training schemes organized on a supra-regional basis. The DHSS, together with the new regional health authorities, is in the process of creating the training posts needed for linking to this scheme. Another possible method might be by the taking up of an appointment in an academic department of community or social medicine and having study leave to participate in the modular courses. Wisely the Faculty has decided not to be too rigid in its attitude towards appropriate training programmes. Furthermore, it is recognized that it is desirable that the specialty should continue to attract persons of maturity from different fields of medical practice, and that such persons may require different educational programmes from those who decide to enter the specialty at an early stage of their postgraduate careers.

The Membership examination will be divided into a first and second part. The first part will examine knowledge in the core subjects of epidemiology, statistics, social sciences in relation to community medicine, and the principles of administration and management. The second part will be designed in such a way as to enable candidates to concentrate on approved work covering a limited number of subjects of their own choosing. The range is wide and, besides involving the core subjects, includes health education, population genetics, health economics, and operational research in relation to health and social services. The presentation of a report on an original project and an oral examination on the subject of the material and related subjects will be required.

To summarize, clinical training should continue for at least one year, and probably two or more, after full registration and might include experience in general practice. During the subsequent two years of general professional training the doctor may either participate in a full-time, or over a longer period, in a series of modular courses on the core subjects. After the acquisition of Part I of the Membership a further period of three years should be undertaken in approved appointments in administrative, academic, or research fields of community medicine, providing increasing responsibility for defined aspects of the health service prior to the candidates being ready for a consultant post.

RECRUITMENT

Unlike the major specialties of medicine, surgery, or general practice, community medicine needs to recruit relatively few doctors into its ranks each year once the present crisis related to reorganization has been overcome. Nonetheless, it is essential that these doctors are of the right calibre if the specialty is to fulfil its role and command respect. Community medicine specialists are inevitably in positions from which they can influence the development of policy and the allocation and utilization of scarce resources. They meet and work with their clinical colleagues over a wide field and they also have extensive involvement both with their colleagues in other professions, such as social work and education, and with lay members of area and regional health authorities as well as with representatives of local government. In clinical medicine the ability to achieve rapport with patients is important; in community medicine the ability to understand and be understood by clinical and other colleagues is an equally essential attribute.

There is no doubt that medical administration is held in disrepute by some clinicians. After 1948 the medical officer of health suffered from a decrease in his responsibilities and isolation from the hospital and GP aspects of health care. The administrative medical officers at regional hospital board level were in many instances remote if not from their consultant colleagues, certainly from junior medical staff, GPs, and public health doctors. In more recent years, however, great efforts have been made both by medical officers of health and regional hospital board medical officers to remedy these problems and to liaise closely both with each other and with executive councils in order to discuss service planning in relation to the total health service. These efforts, which have also involved a growing number of clinicians in the planning and management process, have certainly increased the latter's understanding of the possible role of the community medicine specialist in the future.

The involvement of consultants and GPs in the district management team will allow those doctors interested in medical administration to participate, for some years and on a part-time basis, in planning and management; in the future, for a small but important minority, this might form a useful entrée to training for the specialty. It is important therefore that some young consultants and GPs get the opportunity to participate in management and that junior hospital doctors and trainees in general practice continue to participate in medical executive committee work in hospital, local medical committee work in general practice, and district and area medical advisory committees within the reorganized service.

Satisfactory recruitment to the specialty also depends on adequate training programmes and a well-defined path of possible career development. The recognition, in 1968, by the Royal Commission on Medical Education of the need for community medicine specialists; the publication of the Hunter Report and the resulting clarification of roles and the establishment of the Faculty in 1972, have already had a beneficial effect on recruitment. The establishment of MSc courses in London and Manchester, and the proposals for postgraduate training which have been described, together with the career structure now available in the reorganized health service, give every reason to believe that the specialty is becoming and will remain attractive.

Community medicine will not be the chosen career for more than a few doctors; but one of the exciting aspects of studying medicine is the great width of choice that exists for postgraduate careers. Doctors have contrasting temperaments and interests, some preferring the more immediate emotional rewards of, say, general practice or acute surgery; others gain satisfaction from working in a more diffuse field, such as community medicine, accepting that clear-cut results for their efforts will materialize normally years later rather than in days or weeks. As in all other specialties, community medicine is likely to develop subspecialties. Opportunities therefore also exist within community medicine itself for people of differing temperaments, skills, and interests.

Medicine, and more particularly the health of the community, cannot be considered in isolation from social factors, both historical and present. Doctors working within this specialty particularly need the help and understanding, not only of their health service colleagues, but also of colleagues in other fields, most notably social work, education, town and country planning, and of those working in central government. Doctors who are going to make a success of careers in community medicine must have a general interest in the well-being of the community, with all its ramifications. They should select community medicine as a positive choice not with the expectation that it will be a theoretical backwater remote from the more acute stresses and demands of clinical medicine. They must be prepared for what will usually be a long-term sense of achievement, compared with the more immediate feelings of achievement in clinical medicine. Finally, they must have a liking for continuing debate, and an understanding that decisions at the end of the day may have to take account of political expediency as well as logical deduction and rational planning. Their ultimate satisfaction will lie in observing, over a period of years, new services developing and old ones being reorganized, while knowing that effective services for clinical colleagues, and hence for patients, have been developed more quickly, efficiently, and in a more co-ordinated manner as a result of their efforts.

CONCLUSIONS

The future of community medicine is irrevocably linked with the structure and organization of the remodelled NHS, and the success or failure of reorganization will profoundly affect the specialty. On the other hand, community medicine specialists will be in a unique position in the new health service to influence success or failure. Reorganization involves two major policies: first, integration and secondly, a restructuring of management.

Integration is a philosophy, not just an administrative rationalization, although its definition is notably absent in documents relating to the recent change. The functional interdependence of the primary care and hospital-based services is formally recognized within the administrative framework of the reorganized service, in recognition of the fact that the continuation of the former tripartite structure placed increasing difficulties in the way of rationalizing the balance between hospital and community care. In recent years there has been a steadily growing community orientation in many specialties, particularly in mental handicap, mental illness, care of the elderly, and care of children. The increasing interest of GPs in hospital medicine and traditional local authority specialties has also been apparent.

The medical officer of health and senior administrative medical officer have been in positions from which they were able to influence these trends and those who have taken up new roles as community physicians should have diminishing difficulty in encouraging clinicians to continue to integrate their services and to plan for the whole community rather than according to fragmented specialty demands. Early hospital discharge schemes work well only when strong supporting community services are available. General practitioner maternity units function correctly only with a strong supporting specialist base. It is accordingly reasonable to anticipate that integration of the health service will take place satisfactorily.

Looking further into the future of community medicine inevitably leads one to consider the major problems confronting the NHS, fields where the community medicine specialist is in the best position to help and where he will be personally affected by the success or failure of reorganization.

Basically, the NHS needs to improve the quality of care to individual patients. Many of our foreign colleagues speak of the Service as if it were simply a scheme of 'socialized medicine': health care for the poor, with extensive private practice running in parallel. This, of course, is incorrect but the price to pay for attempting to provide equality of care for all social classes has been a smaller amount of professional time than many patients feel they require and, indeed, than doctors would like to give. A careful look by the community physician, together with his clinical colleagues, at need versus demand will be one of his many new responsibilities. Doctors are the major dispensers of resources within the NHS and the need to rationalize the use of existing resources has led to the proposals to include both GPs and hospital specialists in district management teams.

Clinicians are busy people and the community physician will be a key figure in ensuring, together with his other full-time administrative colleagues, that clinicians' time is not wasted in their new involvement in management and planning. A wide range of clinicians will be needed to participate in health care planning teams. As has been explained, it is known from experience in new town planning that this approach is an appropriate one; for it gives the people responsible for running the service the opportunity to plan and develop it. Such participation can be very rewarding for the clinician. The work involved in interpreting clinical observation into planning proposals is substantial and the community physician at district level, together with the specialists in child health and social service liaison at area level, will need to offer both their time and their skills if health care planning teams are to be viable.

Prevention is a subject in which a growing number of clinicians are now interested, and the development of preventive services will be one of the specific responsibilities of area health authorities. Community physicians will be involved with their clinical colleagues in most aspects of this work: primary prevention in the form of organization of immunization programmes, secondary prevention in the form of screening activities, and tertiary prevention in helping the specialists and GPs to organize continuing care for patients who need it. Health education will be another of the challenges facing community physicians, usually working with specialist health education officers, backed by multidisciplinary teams.

Other difficulties within the NHS stand out as key ones to be tackled in the near future. First, there is the rationalization of general practice. The continuing problem, especially in urban areas, of small single-handed or two-doctor practices makes integration a difficult concept to achieve. The practices tend to be too small and to have inadequate accommodation for attached nursing staff. They are seldom in a position to absorb local authority child health and school health services on a rational basis, as the overlap between adjacent practices is usually extensive. Similarly they are rarely able to work closely with the hospital or to collect the morbidity and other data that would be helpful to the health care planning teams. The community physician cannot change this situation (that will come only from the GPs themselves) but he can facilitate change. Help in planning and building health centres and help with rationalization of medical records are just two ways in which links can be forged.

Occupational health is another service with which the community physician will often find himself concerned. It is not part of the NHS, but the former local health authorities commonly provided occupational health services for local government employees, whereas the hospital service has been remarkably slow in organizing facilities for its own staff. Community physicians, being interested in prevention as well as cure, are likely to become increasingly involved in the rational development and organization of such services.

There are also the important former local authority services of child and school health. The Sheldon Committee (19) made recommendations about the future of the first of these as far back as 1968, but the suggestion that the child health service should gradually be absorbed into general practice has materialized only to a limited extent. There are probably two main reasons for this. First many GPs are not trained in the skills of developmental assessment and, secondly, providing this service is time consuming. The community physicians responsible for child health services in area health authorities will have to review this question and try to determine whether the present methods of organizing the service are really the most efficient and effective, while maintaining the present system for the foreseeable future.

This is in no way a comprehensive list of the scope of the interests and work of the community physician but may give some indication of the potential width and variety of his or her job.

ENVOI

Practitioners of community medicine have now begun to take up their posts in the reorganized NHS. They have come from backgrounds of public health or of hospital medical administration with very few having had experience in both fields; they thus have much to learn, although they already have much to contribute. My plea is that the practitioners of this new specialty should not make undue claims for their abilities and that, on the other side, their clinical colleagues should exercise tolerance and give them time to establish and develop their new roles. If this is done, I have no doubt that within a decade the initial fruits of the work of community physicians will be apparent; and on them they will be willing to be judged.

REFERENCES

1. Royal Commission on Medical Education (1968). *Report 1965–68*, Cmnd. 3703 (London: HMSO).
2. Reid, J. J. A. (1964). 'Future of public health', *Br. med. J.* 2, 1483.
3. —— (1968). *Evolving Practice. In NHS—20th Anniversary Conference* (London: HMSO).
4. Hockey, L. (1966). *Feeling the Pulse* (London: Queen's Institute of District Nursing).
5. Ministry of Health (1968). *The Administrative Structure of the Medical and Related Services in England and Wales* (London: HMSO).
6. Department of Health and Social Security (1970). *The Future Structure of the National Health Service* (London: HMSO).
7. —— (1971). *National Health Service Reorganization. Consultative Document* (London: HMSO).
8. —— (1972). *Report of the Working Party on Medical Administrators* (London: HMSO).
9. —— (1972). *Management Arrangements for the Reorganized National Health Service* (London: HMSO).
10. Scottish Home and Health Department (1971). *Doctors in an Integrated Health Service* (Edinburgh: HMSO).
11. Morris, J. N. (1969). 'Tomorrow's community physician', *Lancet*, ii, 811.
12. Elliott, R. W. (1970). *The Community Physician* (London: County Councils Association).
13. Gooding, D. G., Reid, J. J. A., and Yule, I. G. (1970). 'The community physician's work', *Lancet*, i, 711.
14. de Monchaux, J., *et al.* (1969). 'Milton Keynes: A joint approach to planning', *Br. med. J.* 1, 628.
15. Gooding, D. G., and Reid, J. J. A. (1970). 'Health service planning in new towns', *Med. Offr*, 123, 177.
16. Medical Planning Group (1968). *A Health Service for Milton Keynes, Report* (Aylesbury).
17. Joint Working Party (1974). *Organization of Medical Work in Hospitals, Third Report of Joint Working Party* (London: HMSO).
18. 'Training for specialists in community medicine' (1973). *Faculty Newsletter*, 1, 1, 8.
19. Ministry of Health (1967). *Child Welfare Centres: Report of the Sub-Committee* (London: HMSO).

What price the old firm? or The future of hospital practice

R. L. HIMSWORTH

R. L. HIMSWORTH
MD, MRCP
Research Physician

What price the old firm?
or
The future of hospital practice

INTRODUCTION

In 1974 the first major reform of the NHS was accomplished. This reform, however, was almost exclusively concerned with the administration of the Service. Its initiation went unnoticed by the community at large, by all patients and by most nurses and doctors in hospitals and most GPs. It did not affect the practice of medicine and it was not intended to do so at the outset. Yet medicine has changed greatly since the inception of the NHS in 1948. Indeed, unnoticed by its planners, a Service organized to treat disease was introduced in the middle of a period when the general health of the nation was improving faster than ever before. Although in the popular view medical progress was, and still is, punctuated by 'breakthroughs', this betterment was largely due to unspectacular improvements in social circumstances especially welfare, housing and sanitation, nutrition and preventive medicine. Nowadays, with the single exception of sickness associated with bad habits like smoking, the preventable diseases are mostly prevented and the curable diseases are mostly cured; yet, contrary to the expectations of its originators, the Service becomes more expensive year by year. This phenomenon of the rising cost of health care has occurred in all countries. No matter how the rise is assessed it cannot continue indefinitely whatever the economic situation and prospects of the country. The only ways in which the cost of health can be contained are by a greater degree of efficiency in the use of resources or a diminution in either the quality or the availability of the service. The two latter alternatives are not likely to be advocated or to commend themselves to the public. There will therefore be an increasing call for efficiency. But what is efficiency in this context? Professor A. L. Cochrane in his random reflections on the health service has shown how difficult it is to draw up a balance sheet of cost and benefit in social terms. This being so a cruder yardstick will be used and the object will be to slow or stop the real rise in the expenditure on health care. This process will inevitably entail decisions on priorities and the deployment of resources and consequently changes in the practice of clinical medicine. As approximately three-fifths of the money available for health is spent on the hospitals it is likely that the greatest changes will occur in this part of the Service. In this essay I should like to consider the manner in which doctors in hospitals have become accustomed to look after patients and to use the facilities at their disposal; being a physician my examples are taken from medical practice but the problems are common to all disciplines. The medical profession has given little thought to how it has come to practise medicine as it does and not much more to how it may have to work and organize itself in the future. The next reform of the NHS will surely require more than the modest adjustment of professional attitudes needed in 1974.

Evolution of hospital practice

> Things in themselves new will yet be apprehended with reference to what is old. FRANCIS BACON

The National Health Service Act which came into force in July 1948 contained one major innovation which has been the principal determinant of the hospital service in this country during the last twenty-six years. Instead of the hospitals being under the control of the local authorities, as had been envisaged by the Willink Scheme of 1945 and all the preceding plans, the hospitals were instead nationalized and administered by regional hospital boards, or boards of governors in the case of teaching hospitals, both of which were appointed by the Minister of Health. Only in this way did Mr Aneurin Bevan feel that the maldistribution of hospital facilities, their uneven quality, and the variable size and wealth of the local authorities could all eventually be overcome. A unified hospital service was thus created which was one component of a tripartite administrative structure and which was quite separate from the GP and the residual local authority medical services.

The salaried hospital service which came into being in 1948 and the subsequent introduction in 1953 of the compulsory pre-registration year together with the expansion of the new registrar grade all made it possible for the first time for a substantial number of doctors to have a career exclusively in hospital practice. Over the same time the GPs, who had retained their independence, were given few opportunities to continue to work in hospitals. The cleavage of professional responsibility for patients, which became formalized at this time, had, however, been evolving throughout the first half of the century.

The process was well started when, with the National Insurance Act of 1911, the government first intervened in the financing of general medical care. This Act adopted the 'panel' system of general practice which had been favoured by the Friendly Societies and which was based on payment by capitation charges rather than by item of service. The Act did not cover hospital care. There was thus no incentive for the doctors in such practices to be associated with the charity hospitals which took in their patients. These hospitals were in any case usually teaching hospitals, the staff of which jealously guarded their privileges and access to the hospital facilities. At this time the only free, or nearly free, care available to the dependents of the 'panel' patients was given by the charity hospital out-patient departments. The well-endowed teaching hospitals favoured these out-patient clinics as they provided material for the students. The hospitals for their part undertook the care of the unemployed and the chronic sick who became regular attenders. The out-patient habit, thus encouraged, developed, and was hardened by social circumstances.

The teaching hospital clinics and wards, and also those of the many small hospitals which specialized in diseases of particular systems, were supervised by honorary consultants who by custom gave their services free. This tradition was born of charity but an appointment to the honorary staff was both an indication of professional esteem and a discreet, and permissible, form of advertising. The idea thus became firmly implanted in the minds of many patients and medical students that 'hospital doctors' were better able to deal with serious disease. The middle classes, however, still paid their family doctors for their services and a second opinion was obtained by seeing a specialist in his rooms or summoning him to the bedside. Although there was a system of private nursing homes and local cottage hospitals many patients were treated, and even operated upon, in their own homes. (This old tradition flowed into the spring of modern surgery when in 1951 a thoracotomy and lung resection was done in a makeshift operating theatre in Buckingham Palace.)

At the end of the First World War the importance of health matters was recognized by the creation of a Ministry of Health which was conceived and headed by the first, and so far only, medically qualified minister. The next decade was punctuated by a succession of neglected reports which did nothing for a deteriorating situation. It was not until 1929 and the Local Government Act that any major changes occurred. This Act led to the administrative but not physical reconstruction of the hospitals previously run under the old Poor Laws. These public general hospitals had salaried medical staffs but there were few senior posts, promotion was slow and consequently there was little enthusiasm in the profession for the jobs. The GPs at this time attempted to obtain 'hospital privileges' in these institutions but for the most part they failed. Visiting consultants, who did not have charge of beds, were, however, engaged to supplement the work of the whole-time staff in the local authority hospitals. These consultants were paid well for their services.

The decade of the 1930s was one of haphazard progress throughout the country but all was disrupted by the war. The Emergency Medical Service showed that central country-wide administration was possible and paved the way for a unified hospital service. And the National Health Service Act followed. It should, however, be noted that the Minister responsible faced with the opposition of the local authorities and the medical profession split the latter and overcame the former. The honorary consultants were to be rewarded for the work they had previously done for nothing and in exchange they yielded none of their freedom but dropped their opposition to the Act. The GPs gave up all but their last toeholds in the hospitals but remained as independent contractors. The local authorities lost the hospitals.

What were these hospitals like? It is astonishing to read that of the hospitals which the NHS took over 70 per cent had fewer than one hundred beds and 30 per cent less than thirty. From the outset the objective was to eliminate these small units. Two years before the Act Mr Bevan proclaimed: 'I would rather be kept alive in the efficient if cold altruism of a large hospital than expire in a gush of warm sympathy in a small one.' Since 1962, but even before then, the district hospital has been the ideal with its staff of consultants able to cope with all but the most complex disease situations. It is the major achievement of the NHS that the country is now covered by a sufficiency of such institutions. Although much is now being written of the persisting uneven distribution of medical facilities, nevertheless it is true that across the country the standard of hospital care for acute illness is among the best in the world. But the attainment of this standard has brought problems and its maintenance will bring others. The greatest of these future problems is staff of all grades, but I shall be concerned in this essay only with the medical staffing.

When the district hospitals were created by amalgamation and expansion of the existing facilities, and even on occasion by building new hospitals, consultants were appointed in the various specialties. These individuals had, of course, been trained in teaching hospitals where they were familiar with the 'firm' system of apprenticeship and delegation of clinical responsibility. Furthermore the majority had done military service where their respectful deference, even a characteristic of the medical profession, had become hardened into an acceptance of an hierarchical system. These consultants insisted on the adoption without adaptation of the familiar stereotype of practice within the teaching hospital. The full panoply of the firm system was unfolded and displayed: my beds, my ward, my out-patients, my houseman and, a little later, my registrar. But if all this was necessary, and none questioned that it was, is it still needed? Indeed will it be possible to maintain this system?

The first twenty years

It is very difficult to determine whether hospitals function efficiently. Some of the crude statistics for the first twenty years of the NHS have been assembled in Table 1. During this period there were only minor changes in the expectation of life of any age-group of either sex and the death-rate fluctuated but little. In crude life and death terms therefore the NHS had little effect. There was, however, a rise in both the population and in absence from work due to sickness. The number of occupied beds in hospital fell steadily during the second half of the period but they were used more intensively. The number of professional staff (nurses and doctors) employed in the hospitals doubled.

TABLE I

The first twenty years of the National Health Service. Population, numbers of doctors, and hospital administrative statistics: England and Wales

	1949	*1959*	*1969*
Population	43,785,000	45,386,000	48,827,000
Deaths per 1,000	11·7	11·6	11·9
General practitioners	—	22,091	21,505
Consultants*	3,488	5,322	7,763
SHMO and medical assistants	1,106	1,530	1,124
Senior registrars	1,430	931	1,431
Registrars and JHMOs	1,924	3,460	4,489
Senior house officers	797	2,315	4,761
House officers	2,613	2,436	2,405
Nurses	137,636	190,946	262,644
Beds occupied daily ($\times 10^3$)	398	413	380
Discharges and deaths ($\times 10^3$)	2,937	4,000	5,282
New out-patients ($\times 10^3$)	6,148	7,235	8,055
Out-patient follow-up visits ($\times 10^3$)	19,853	21,811	25,335

*Whole-time equivalents. In 1969 there were 9,431 doctors with consultant contracts.

Looking at the medical staffing more closely it can be seen that the number of house officers (mostly provisionally registered doctors) did not change during the first twenty years of the NHS but the number of consultants more than doubled. This does not indicate any breakdown in the 'firm' system but reflects the increased numbers of consultants in specialties where house officers are unusual (for example, pathology and anaesthetics). In England in 1972 there were in general medicine more house officers than consultants and almost equal numbers of SHOs and registrars (senior and junior) and consultants. The British general medical firm therefore usually consists of a consultant, a registrar, an SHO, and a houseman. Table 1 also shows that efforts to establish a sub-consultant grade (SHMO or medical assistant) with an ambiguous relationship to the 'firm' have been unsuccessful.

As is well known, the major expansions in the grades of hospital doctors have been at the top and in the intermediate grades. In England and Wales the equivalent of more than 4,000 new consultant posts and 6,500 new registrar jobs were created at an average rate of over 500 a year. This expansion, together with the loss of doctors by death, retirement, or emigration and the meagre output of doctors by the medical schools, made it inevitable that the Service should become increasingly dependent upon foreign medical graduates. Even though this has long been recognized as a bad thing the trend has not been halted. In 1963, 42 per cent of all registrars and 54 per cent of all senior house officers in England and Wales were born outside the United Kingdom and Ireland. In 1971 the figures were 56 and 59 per cent, respectively.

TABLE 2

General medicine: hospital medical staff: England

	1963	*1972*
Consultants*	553 (736)	777 (936)
Senior registrars	104	144
Registrars	499	586
Senior house officers	318	717
House officers	1,039	990
All staff	2,602	3,252

*Whole-time equivalents, actual number of consultants is shown in parentheses.

If the medical staff has been increasing in numbers and the number of patients treated by hospitals has also been going up what has been happening to the workload of the doctors? It is difficult to make any but the crudest of estimates. Let us, however, consider the 'specialty' of general medicine in England in the early 1960s and again ten years later; excluded from consideration are those branches of medicine which require a disproportionately large number of doctors to patients (for example, nephrology, cardiology, neurology), those in which the work is mostly in out-patient clinics (for example, dermatology, venereology) and those like paediatrics and geriatrics which are separated organizationally from general medicine. Table 2 shows the numbers and type of doctor employed and Table 3 the work they did. If these data are combined some idea of the annual work of an average general medical 'firm' can be obtained. If there is one house officer to a firm it can be estimated that the average daily number of in-patients on a firm was constant at about 27 and that the number of patients admitted under the firm in the course of a year rose during the decade from 530 to 700. This rise of 32 per cent was matched by a 25 per cent increase in the number of medical staff. Thus more efficient use of beds does not mean that the physicians are working any harder. It might be argued that more was being done for these patients during their shorter stay in hospital and the rapid increase in the use of investigational facilities is often used to support this argument. It is more difficult to show that intense investigative evaluation makes more patients better more quickly. Turning to the situation in out-patient clinics, and assuming that all new referrals are seen by a consultant or registrar, it can be calculated that the average number of new patients seen by each doctor each week fell from 9·0 in the early 1960s to 6·5 in 1972. Likewise, on the assumption that all members of the firm saw follow-ups in the clinic the number seen per week by each doctor fell slightly from 17 to 16. The work of the average medical firm does not appear to be unduly arduous.

TABLE 3

General medicine: patients cared for: England

	Thousands	
	1962	*1972*
Beds: average occupied daily	28·5	26·2
Discharges and deaths	552	692
New out-patients	584	518
Out-patient follow-ups	2,305	2,686

The data in Table 3 show that the numbers of admissions to general medical beds increased by 25 per cent during a period when the adult population increased by only 6 per cent. As the over-all indices of health (for example, mortality, morbidity) show no change over this time and as the average length of stay in hospital for this category of patient fell from 18·9 to 13·9 days, it can only be concluded that not only was more effective treatment being given but also that diseases which were previously treated in the home were more commonly being admitted to hospital. The development of more effective forms of treatment does not inevitably mean that a corresponding increase in medical sophistication is necessary to apply them. During the period in question medical practice in and out of hospital has altered radically with the introduction of psychotropic drugs and diuretic agents to give but two examples. If the trend continues will the medical firm with its pinnacle of experience buttressed by junior staff be the most appropriate organizational unit of the future?

The discussion so far has focused on the firm but this in turn is centred on the consultant. What does he do? One of the curious features of the NHS is the blurring of the distinction between a 'consultant' and a 'specialist'. Most consultant physicians in district hospitals are generalists with a special interest. They do not as a rule treat solely one category of patient and usually their patients will have a wide range of disorders. The great majority of these patients probably do not even need a consultant's, let alone a specialist's opinion and for this reason can be quite satisfactorily managed in out-patient departments by registrars in training without reference to the chief. The consultant will, however, regularly see the patients in his beds although he may not intervene in their treatment. The special expertise of these doctors is most often fully utilized only when they are asked to see patients by their colleagues or when teaching their juniors. Even within teaching hospitals most of the staff are biased generalists rather than specialists. It has been a failure of the NHS that it has not used well the gradation of ability and experience within the consultant grade and that the tendency has been to level down.

In this first half of the essay I have tried to show how the pattern of the general physician's work in and out of hospital has developed; how it has evolved in response to social and community pressures almost wholly external to medicine; and how the firm system has been adopted and amplified. I should now like to turn to the factors which will mould medical practice in the next two decades.

The future pressures from without

The forces which will determine the shape of medical practice within the NHS in the future are three: the application of technology and research, the facilities which will be made available, and lastly the number and quantity of the medical staff.

TECHNOLOGY AND RESEARCH

It may seem extraordinary to consider medical research and technology as external forces for change. The Health Service, however, is not innovative and has developed no mechanisms for the systematic evaluation and incorporation of medical knowledge into its planning. On the other hand the medical profession itself is collectively conservative whilst at the same time allowing full rein to individual enthusiasms. Some examples should suffice to make this point clear.

First consider two success stories. Less than forty years ago it became possible, by mechanical means, to maintain the breathing of patients with acute respiratory failure which was, in those days, usually due to poliomyelitis. A generous benefaction provided hospitals up and down the country with the necessary equipment. In the following twenty years the polio virus was isolated and cultured and vaccines were prepared from it. The community was generally immunized, the disease virtually disappeared from the country and the machinery became redundant. Again, in 1948 there were 26,000 hospital beds used for the treatment (by rest) of tuberculosis. Coincidentally effective therapy (streptomycin) was developed. Fortunately this antibiotic was not made available to doctors until it had been properly evaluated by the first large-scale therapeutic trials for there is no doubt that the profession left to itself would have misused both this drug and its successors. Even today after all the immaculately conceived and executed clinical trials on the chemotherapy of tuberculosis the variation in modes of therapy and surveillance of patients can only be ascribed to the freedom and idiosyncrasy of medical practice.

But if these are success stories what is more usual? The typical precipitant of death these days is the summation of an acute episode on a slowly evolving but well-established chronic pathological state. Much modern medicine is an attempt to cover the acute event. All doctors are taught about ischaemic heart disease but the story, which is still unfolding, of methods of treating an acute myocardial infarct is at least as illuminating and even more educative. Controversy swirls whilst practice lags. What is the optimum period of rest? What were the real costs of the anti-coagulant fashion and were there any benefits? At present the expensive enthusiasm for coronary care units is barely contained by administrative and financial considerations and not at all by the lack of evidence that they have a major effect on the over-all mortality. But these units do highlight certain facets of the application of technology to the treatment of medical conditions.

Characteristically technology has been applied to single organ failures: chronic dialysis and transplantation for kidney disease, cardiac monitoring and pacemaking are good examples. The technology used is not intended to affect the evolution of the underlying pathological condition; it is not therefore concerned with disease but with an established situation. It does not seek to cure. The patient salvaged by medical technology will most probably require medical supervision for the remainder of his life. But even the short-term hopes for the most successful technology are belied by the long-term problems. The first and most benevolent technical innovation in medicine must surely be the use of insulin in the treatment of diabetes mellitus. In retrospect this therapy foreshadowed in miniature all the problems which have now loomed in other fields. The technical difficulties were overcome; suitable insulins were manufactured; patients were taught to inject themselves, to look after their own equipment, and to assess their own condition; special clinics were set up to oversee treatment. But the disease was not cured. Eventually the patient's well-being diminished with the development of the complications of diabetes. We now know that from the outset the expectation of life of these patients is curtailed. Likewise evidence is now accumulating that patients with renal transplants who retain functioning grafts do not have a normal life expectancy but die early from vascular disease. Thus technological expedients are only moderately successful and are very expensive not only in terms of buildings and equipment (special care units with their life-support and monitoring machines and laboratories for controlling treatment) but also in trained staff.

Lewis Thomas is surely justified in talking of 'half-way technology', for the solutions are inherently unimaginative and, being based only on current knowledge, may become, like the old iron lung, rapidly outmoded. The old adage 'prevention is better than cure' seems to be forgotten. Prevention is also cheaper and may follow from social changes. The original impetus to cardiac surgery was the treatment of chronic rheumatic heart disease. The improvement in living conditions during the last thirty years has all but eliminated the antecedent rheumatic fever. Who can say how the pattern of disease in the country might be changed if everyone stopped smoking cigarettes? The solutions to these problems are essentially social and are already attainable.

If prevention is not possible common sense would suggest that the early detection and treatment of asymptomatic disease are the next best thing. But the natural history of chronic disease today is not generally deflected by treatment and, contrary to expectation, early diagnosis may not benefit the patient. Moreover, the technology spawned by mass screening is creating new problems. As more elaborate biochemical and physical tests become possible so it becomes economic to combine them into diagnostic gift packs. Luxuriant and unsolicited information is provided and with the proliferation of results the likelihood of the occurrence of laboratory error or actual abnormality increases. Neither can be neglected but, whilst the former can be excluded by repetition, the significance of the latter might be doubtful. The work involved in allaying such a doubt can be prodigious and the effect on the patient disastrous. The physician of the future will have to be taught to write: 'I have noted this abnormal result and intend to ignore it. The information was not requested and upon reflection it does not throw any light upon the patient's condition.'

So far I have said little about the impact of research on the practice of medicine. In particular I have avoided the banal arena of cancer. An effective treatment for cancer, like any other technical innovation, would throw an increased burden on the available medical facilities. A method of preventing cancer would in all probability have little effect on the need for medical services because, as the late Professor H. R. Dean used to observe, 'the longer you avoid dying of cancer the more likely you are to die of something else' and the majority of deaths from malignancy occur after the age of 60 when the life expectancy is short and the likelihood of the need for medical care is increasing.

A century ago Sir William Gull wrote: 'Decay and death are physiological—that is natural and part of life; but we had rather not think so. We would rather that the course of nature was more in our own hands.' Presidential crusades against cancer, heart disease, and stroke do not indicate an accretion of human wisdom over the years. Fruitful research in the future will surely improve the quality of life by increasing the simplicity and effectiveness of treatment and reducing the morbidity from the less dramatic, non-lethal conditions. Only in the fields of psychiatry and congenital abnormality is the 'course of nature' likely to be significantly changed by research.

The deployment by the NHS of technologically advanced

facilities required only by relatively few patients but needing specialized skills and large staffs will be critical to its future development and will be a major factor in moulding the shape of the hospital system. Special departments have in the past been scattered about: a cardio-thoracic unit in this district hospital, a dialysis unit in that teaching hospital. Although facilities have been provided on a regional basis, the excellence which can only come from a concentration of resources has not been achieved. The usual district hospital is too small to contain more than a single special unit but it is not large enough to afford the full back-up facilities or, if they are provided, they are under-utilized. The teaching hospitals, on the other hand, have not been built up as centres of excellence. The price of a uniformly high plateau of clinical care has been the failure to develop any prominent landmarks on the medical scene. Perhaps the district hospitals will be judged in the future to have been too good for their purpose. The logic of the situation would seem to demand a pyramidal structure with all varieties of specialized and uncommon skills collected into one institution at the apex and a spreading base of hospitals of diminishing sophistication beneath.

HOSPITAL RESOURCES

It is not my intention to discuss in detail the financing of health care. A few general points need to be restated, however, if only because those who work in the NHS often seem to ignore the unbiological instability of the 'milieu intérieur' of the body of the State. The money made available to nourish the Service depends upon two factors: first, the condition of the economy and, second, a political appraisal of the minimum level of medical care which the electorate will accept. This minimum level is substantially above that which the well-being of the community as a whole requires and is apparently rising. Nevertheless, it is lower than in some other comparable countries. But whilst such international comparisons may be interesting they are politically irrelevant when determining the financial allocation for the service. Major economies in running costs of the NHS are difficult to make, for the public would rapidly become aware of a deterioration in standards. Cancellation of major capital expenditure, however, is easy; moreover, it is not thought to generate the same electoral opprobrium even though it demoralizes the staff concerned. The intention to build new hospitals and health centres has therefore been repeatedly given up in order to assuage the vagaries of the economic situation. It is not therefore surprising that only half the beds in the country are in hospitals put up in this century and only about 1·5 per cent of the total in use are being built or replaced each year.

In the last fifty years hospitals have acquired a new function. No longer do they simply care for sick in the wards and in the out-patient departments. They have now become the centre of the diagnostic services in their neighbourhood and these facilities are increasingly being made available to the GPs.

Modern hospitals are expensive both to build and to run and, as has already been noted, they monopolize two-thirds of the financial resources available to the NHS. Hospitals could be used more efficiently. What comparably expensive factory functions eight hours a day, five days a week, with a skeleton staff at all other times? This pattern of use could be defended when extended bed rest was an important part of treatment. But the duration of hospital admission for an acute illness has progressively shortened and the fractional cost of the hospital wards has diminished greatly as the expense of the ancillary departments (laboratories, X-ray equipment, operating theatres) has increased. The case for more efficient use of the existing resources is unanswerable. The solution lies not merely in the 'better use of beds' and deployment of the staff looking after the in-patients, which I shall discuss later, but also in more intensive and imaginative use of the hospital services. Clinics could be held and diagnostic procedures could be carried out in the evenings and at the week-end. (It is interesting to speculate on the real saving to the economy if the work in hospital was reorganized so that no out-patient attended during the working day.) As yet only very timid steps have been taken along this road in this country. The much praised 'five-day' ward is an astonishing example of the primitive economic logic which inspires the administration of the Service.

It is inevitable that some form of 'audit' of the way in which hospital resources are utilized will have to be introduced because in-patient care is the most expensive form of treatment.

MEDICAL STAFFING OF HOSPITALS

That there is a shortage of doctors in the UK has been a notable point of universal agreement ever since the Willink Report suggested that there were too many. Despite the expansion of the number of medical students in the past few years the number of doctors qualifying by the end of the decade will be fewer than even the modest target set by the Royal Commission on Medical Education which reported in 1966. The shortage of doctors will be exacerbated in the immediate future by factors which if not new in themselves will have increased effects. First, there will be proportionately more women doctors for whose special career needs no provision is at present made. Secondly, the uncertainty of the general economic situation and persistent under-financing of the NHS will lead to a new wave of medical emigration. Thirdly, medical immigration which is already diminishing will most probably be further curtailed by the introduction of some test of both professional competence and knowledge of English. The effect of all three factors will first be felt in the junior grades of the hospital service which are already depleted by the developing preference of British medical graduates for general practice.

One minor reform which could be implemented rapidly and would afford some temporary relief from this shortage would be to co-ordinate the starting and terminal dates of all posts in the NHS. At present a significant number of junior doctors are unemployed between jobs. If all house officer jobs began on 1 January and 1 July and all more senior posts on 1 July it would be possible to tailor a course of training to suit an individual without any of the frustrations and periods of uncertainty and idleness which now litter the path of the young hospital doctor.

It seems likely that it will soon be impossible to fill more than a small proportion of the junior, training posts throughout the NHS. The only solution is to change radically the organization of clinical care and the career structure for doctors in hospitals.

A pattern for the future

Let me now for the first time turn to the patient who is, after all, the person the system is supposed to help. And let us follow two patients into and out of hospital.

John S. is 60 and has bronchitis. Over the course of a few days his symptoms become worse until his wife sends for the doctor. The GP when he comes recognizes the familiar acute exacerbation of the underlying chronic condition. He knows that John needs antibiotics and antispasmodics and that a chest X-ray and sputum culture might be helpful. John would probably get well if treated at home but he might become worse. So John's family doctor decides to send him to hospital knowing that physiotherapy and warmth will speed his recovery and that Mrs S. is out at work all day. When John arrives at the hospital he is first seen in the casualty department by the house physician of the firm 'on take' who examines him, orders a chest X-ray, sputum culture, blood count, and a few other tests and finally writes him up for antibiotics, antispasmodics, and physiotherapy. Later that day the registrar also sees John, looks at the X-ray and confirms the prescribed regime. The following day on 'the round' the consultant, the registrar, and the houseman, accompanied by the ward sister and the physiotherapist, all review John's treatment which requires no modification in the light of the laboratory findings. Two rounds and a week later it is decided that John is well enough to go home. This is the only decision taken during the course of John's entire stay in hospital.

Peter D. develops acute chest pain at work and is immediately sent to hospital in an ambulance. An acute myocardial infarct is suspected by the casualty medical officer and confirmed by an electrocardiogram. Over the next few days Peter's condition is perilous. Successive episodes of cardiac arrhythmia are diagnosed and managed individually, heart failure is corrected when it occurs, diabetes mellitus is discovered and assessed. The available resources of the hospital are deployed for Peter's benefit. Houseman, registrar, and consultant singly and together make a series of decisions about Peter's treatment. At the outset things are decided from hour to hour, then from day to day, and finally from round to round until Peter, too, leaves hospital.

It is quite clear that John S. and Peter D. are quite different categories of patient. Both should be in hospital but, while one requires the closest surveillance and frequent active intervention, the other needs only a friendly eye to see that improvement is steady. Incidentally, both John and Peter were seen, as a matter of course, in the out-patient clinic a couple of weeks after they left hospital. Both continued to attend at intervals over the following months although there was no change in their clinical state and therefore no alteration in therapy. Both had also to see their GPs throughout this time because departmental adherence to archaic accounting principles led to the hospital restricting the amount of drugs on out-patient prescriptions to two weeks' supply.

Hopefully things will be done differently in the future. John S. and Peter D. will still need to be in hospital. John because his social circumstances do not allow him to be ill for long at home and because the general expectation in the community will be for illness of his degree to warrant hospital admission. And Peter will still need close medical supervision which will be provided in much the same way as now. But John could be looked after in a very different fashion. In years to come John's family doctor having assessed his condition would send him up to hospital together with his case-notes which would set out the problem and how he would like John to be treated. John would be admitted straight to the ward where the ward sister, by now invested with a responsibility compatible with her training and experience, would arrange for the doctor's instructions to be carried out. John's doctor would come in briefly and as necessary to assess his progress and, together with the sister, would decide when John could go home. In the ordinary way there would be no need for John to be seen by a house physician or registrar, but should he not improve then a consultant could be asked to see him either by his family doctor or by the ward sister. The consultant would not take over but would act as an adviser giving a specialist opinion. Nevertheless consultants on the staff of a hospital would be charged with a general responsibility for the welfare of patients and the efficient running of the hospital. They would be allowed to override the decisions of GPs about in-patients in the same way as they can now over-rule the actions of their registrars and housemen. This necessarily involves the recognition by the profession that the practice of medicine now requires the scrupulously non-interventionist etiquette of the past to be discarded in favour of a more flexible but equally courteous convention. Furthermore in giving senior nurses on the wards more scope to use their judgement their work would be both more interesting and more important than that of their administrative sisters. It is worth remembering at this point that one group of doctors, obstetricians, habitually and happily delegate a very large proportion of their clinical work to midwives.

As we have seen, GPs have never had 'hospital privileges' in this country. All doctors under our system get the same training until they are fully registered as medical practitioners. Doctors whose careers are spent in hospitals are not better, they just work differently. There is therefore no question that the GPs are capable of this kind of hospital work. The population is largely concentrated into towns and the family doctors practising within the immediate vicinity of the district hospital which admits their patients already find time to visit them in hospital. For a large part of this country, therefore, there would be no logistic difficulties if the family physicians continued to look after the majority of their patients in hospital.

How would Peter D. with his infarct or Jane W. with her overdose fare under such a system? It is clear that the category of patients who require frequent decisions about their treatment need to be admitted to a ward for medical emergencies. Here the junior staff (reduced in numbers because they do not look after all the general medical patients in the hospital) will be concentrated. Here they will work under the direction of the consultant on call for that day in an acute ward which will combine the functions, now dispersed, of observation ward, intensive care unit, coronary care unit, and the acute aspect of the present medical wards. This group of doctors will, of course, be available to deal with unexpected medical crises elsewhere in the hospital, and a patient with, for example, a post-operative pulmonary embolism could be moved to their unit for close supervision. This method of organizing hospital work depends upon the proportion of cases requiring frequent decisions about treatment. Most probably about one-fifth of the general medical admissions to hospital fall into this category.

A further advantage of this mode of hospital organization would be an improved system for higher medical training. The junior staff appointments could be made at regional level and with co-ordination of the dates of appointment a proper postgraduate training scheme extending over several years and with rotation through different departments of various types of hospital could easily be organized. The non-educative chores of medicine would be reduced and a proper balance between teaching and apprenticeship restored.

What about the out-patient clinics? They should be abolished and the money saved used to build and service health centres. Just as it is easy for general practitioners to visit their local hospital, so it should be easy for a consultant to do his out-patient work in the health centre by monthly or weekly visits. A free professional interchange would be facilitated, a single set of notes could be kept about each patient and there would be no need to write letters. (In some parts of China patients keep their own notes and produce them for the doctor. It is an attractive thought.) As now the laboratory and investigative facilities of the hospital could be used: blood samples could be taken to the hospital from the health centre and only if elaborate tests were needed would the patient have to go to the hospital.

The consultant would thus be freed to use his professional skills and special expertise. A more rational use of junior staff would allow their numbers to be reduced and their career prospects improved. The interest and satisfaction of the GPs' life would increase although the number of patients on their lists might have to be reduced. Probably it would also be necessary to rationalize and bring together the various specialist units now scattered through the hospitals, creating in effect centres of excellence which would be the focal point not only of the hospital system in the regions but also of the postgraduate training programmes.

These ideas are not new. They are much the same as those put forward more than fifty years ago in the Dawson Report on the future provision of medical services. Then the ideas were welcomed both by the public at large and the profession but the impetus to reform ran out in the sands of political distraction and economy. Soon the impetus will come again and will be sustained by the twin external forces of economic necessity and shortage of doctors. It is to be hoped that the need for change will be recognized by the whole medical community and that the profession will take the lead in the next reorganization of the NHS.

Conclusion

Every craft evolves its own way of working. Whilst this evolution proceeds in step with the erection of the framework within which the profession functions all is well but, if the frame changes faster than professional attitudes, then stresses are set up. Restrictive practices, demarcation disputes, over-manning: these are the sociological terms for some of the symptoms of such stresses. The symptoms are manifest in the community of doctors. Old professional divisions have become outmoded as new skills have become widely distributed, as the pattern of illness has changed, and as the organization of medical care has developed. The greatest and most long-standing of these divisions is between the doctors who work in hospitals and the GPs. It need not exist, indeed it must not persist. The logic of the situation requires that the present distinctions should be blurred and merged into a continuum of co-operative care for patients.

SOURCES

I have not given references in the course of the text. The figures in the tables are all derived from *Health and Personal Social Services Statistics for England and Wales 1972* and for England 1973. I have also used the Report of the Royal Commission on Medical Education 1965–8. I have drawn from three illuminating books: *The Hospitals 1800–1948* by Professor Brian Abel-Smith (Heinemann, 1964); *The Changing National Health Service* by R. G. S. Brown (Routledge & Kegan Paul, 1973); and *Effectiveness and Efficiency: Random Reflections on Health Services* by Professor A. L. Cochrane (Nuffield Provincial Hospitals Trust, 1972). To all who have not read it may I recommend Dr Lewis Thomas's essay 'The technology of medicine' in *The New England Journal of Medicine*, 285 (1971), 1366. The quotation from Francis Bacon may be found in 'Aphorisms', Book 1 of *The New Organon* and that from Sir William Gull is in a collection of his published writings (The New Sydenham Society, 1896).

The place and relationships of the chest service and chest diseases within the National Health Service

ROSEMARY MULLIGAN

ROSEMARY MULLIGAN
BSc, MD, MRCP
General physician with an interest in chest disease

The place and relationships of the chest service and chest diseases within the National Health Service

The chest services in the past have occupied a unique position in the health care of this country through being dominated by the problems of a single preventable disease: tuberculosis. Its detection in symptomatic patients and their asymptomatic contacts, its treatment with the limited tools of the time and the removal and isolation of infectious cases from the general environment started the decline in its incidence before chemotherapy became widely available. Close links with local health authorities necessarily developed and the isolation sanatorium for long-term care played a key role. Two types of chest specialists evolved: the one whose work was concerned solely with pulmonary tuberculosis, commonly employed by the local authority and called tuberculosis officers, the other whose general medical interests within the general hospital showed a preference for respiratory disease and who therefore as a matter of course became concerned also with the care of pulmonary tuberculosis.

With the decline of the disease, many tuberculosis officers widened their sphere of interest to concern themselves with other respiratory diseases as well. This process clearly depended on the part of the country involved because of marked variation in the incidence of tuberculosis and the greater problems presented by the disease in the towns.

Tuberculosis dispensaries disappeared but chest clinics continued, often totally geographically separate from the general hospital whose administration they shared. Even when situated within a general hospital the organization, including medical records, staff and radiological facilities were separate from those of the rest of the hospital. Links with the local authority remained close and larger clinics employed full-time health visitors whose main task was contact tracing and regular visiting of those patients on the tuberculosis register.

The decline of tuberculosis was brought about by a combination of case detection through mass radiography units and subsequent isolation, through BCG vaccination and the advent of effective chemotherapy. In 1947, there were 43,159 notifications and 20,156 deaths from respiratory tuberculosis. In 1965, the figures were 13,552 and 2,008, respectively. The decline in number of deaths has continued and deaths from all forms of tuberculosis in 1971 reached 1,438. The proportion of deaths to notifications also continues to fall. It is salutary, however, to realize that tuberculosis still causes more deaths than any other notifiable infectious disease in England and Wales. Even more astonishing are the findings of the British Thoracic and Tuberculosis Association Research Committee which examined all death certificates in which tuberculosis appeared in 1968 and succeeded in investigating two-thirds of them through local chest physicians. A proportion showed no evidence of tuberculosis on closer scrutiny. One-quarter of those certified as dying of tuberculosis had in fact died of the late effects of tuberculous scarring such as respiratory failure. The shaming fact that approximately one-fifth of those with active tuberculosis were diagnosed after death at post-mortem examination, and that one-third of the active cases had been given inadequate chemotherapy by modern standards speaks for itself. The Committee makes the point that where failures occurred, they were due to failure to adhere to generally accepted standard practice. The changing pattern of the disease in this country has and will continue to require modification of the approach to its control. Hopefully the 10 per cent annual decline in incidence of respiratory tuberculosis will continue or even increase.

With the decline of tuberculosis and the very real possibility of its virtual eradication in this country, many forecast the end to the need for chest clinics in the future and even for the necessity of specialists in chest diseases at all. Whereas the former has become accepted as right and indeed inevitable, the latter has proved far from reality.

With the decline of tuberculosis, the relative importance of other respiratory diseases has increased. Many notable advances have been made in the understanding of a number of pulmonary diseases and their management in the past ten to fifteen years. With the broadening of the interest of chest physicians, has come greater involvement in respiratory problems of systemic diseases in general hospitals, and the training needs for future specialists have required review.

The rapid decline in incidence of tuberculosis was recognized in the late 1950s and the future of the chest services was examined by the Standing Tuberculosis Advisory Committee in 1960. The main proposals were that the chest physician should be a member of staff of a general hospital, that the chest clinic should be integrated into the out-patient department of the hospital where feasible and that chest physicians should continue to manage tuberculosis as a primary duty. The report of the committee set up by the Central Health Services Council, under the chairmanship of Professor J. G. Scadding, took these proposals further, so that it was recommended for example that the chest physician should also undertake a share of general medical work, junior posts in general medicine being a necessary part of his training. It was accepted that a chest department should be incorporated into the facilities of any general hospital, special accommodation being unnecessary and should be staffed as should any other specialty. Thoracic units were seen as sited in major centres with facilities for more complex investigations and thoracic surgery, serving areas up to regional size. The need for pure chest specialists for major centres was acknowledged, as was the need for special experience in tuberculosis for all chest physicians.

This report has been used as a guide for subsequent development of the chest services and its proposals have been widely implemented. Numerous small chest clinics have been closed, and those existing within general hospitals or geographically near them have been absorbed into the general hospital services. Separate secretarial records and radiological facilities have in many places disappeared. Experience of this transition has been favourable.

It proved difficult, however, to predict career prospects in the specialty. The chest clinic organization was contracting but, countering this, medical assistants and senior hospital medical officers were being phased out on retirement and general physicians with an interest in chest diseases were being appointed, who would spend a large part of their time on the general rather than chest work. Furthermore, 70 per cent of consultants in the specialty were found to be over 50 years of age.

The reports of the Joint Tuberculosis Committee of the British Thoracic and Tuberculosis Association and the Committee on Thoracic Medicine (Royal College of Physicians, London) drew attention to these facts in 1971 and also to the facts that twelve consultant posts should be expected to fall vacant annually, which would require 48 senior registrars in training, including those on rotating appointments, with a minimum of 24 doing the thoracic part of the rotation. In 1961 there were only 8 senior registrar posts in thoracic medicine. Expansion of these training posts was recommended as a matter of urgency and a number of such posts have been created. The crisis in staffing of chest departments has thus been largely met by the increase in the senior registrar establishment.

As regards the diseases with which the chest physician of the future will have to cope, it is worth noting first that respiratory diseases form the largest group of diseases seen in general practice. Deaths from respiratory diseases as a whole in England and Wales have remained very much the same over the last twenty years, at around 90,000 a year, with slight peaks during some winters due to the acute respiratory infections such as influenza. It is the pattern of the diseases within this number that have shown marked changes. First of all tuberculosis which, although contained, is not yet controlled and could be eradicated. The age at which most tuberculosis occurs has changed from the young to the old, peak rates occurring in males over 65 years. The urban incidence of the disease remains higher than the rural incidence. One survey revealed that Indian-born and Pakistan-born persons had twelve times and twenty-six times, respectively, the rate of tuberculous infection of those British born.

Non-respiratory tuberculosis is common in these groups. Immigrants therefore form a high-risk group and doctors should consider tuberculosis (often atypical) in any obscure illness in immigrant races. The case for Heaf testing and giving BCG to immigrant children at an early age has often been made.

The value of follow-up of patients with tuberculous scarring has been called into question. These patients constituted the bulk of the huge chest clinics of the past. In order to accommodate other problems in the out-patients it would be necessary to continue to cut down drastically on their attendances. Radiological changes in this group are often not evident until the patient is symptomatic, and annual sputum examination would be of more value than a chest X-ray in the patient with extensively scarred lungs. Treatment with chemotherapy of all patients with extensive scarring would prevent some reactivations but would be costly and as a large-scale measure, would probably be impracticable. Large numbers of these follow-ups need not continue but the patient should be warned to report suspicious symptoms so that GPs can send the patient either to an open access radiological session at the general hospital for an X-ray or refer him back to the out-patients. Referrals of patients with symptoms to mass radiography units by GPs has been found to yield a higher proportion of active tuberculous cases than random surveys of the population.

Operations for tuberculosis are now rare and the patients with grossly scarred lungs, with scars from phrenic crush operations and thorocoplasties are dying out. As regards patients who have had the standard chemotherapy for eighteen months or two years, initially with three drugs: any follow-up of these is now considered unnecessary once chemotherapy has ceased. The only difficulty here is to be certain that the drugs have been consumed. This will become less of a problem in future because of the more widespread use of the second-line drugs where patient acceptance is likely to be better. The long-term effectiveness of short regimes of treatment with the newer drugs have yet to be evaluated and the virtual certainty of cure with streptomycin, PAS, and INAH taken for two years cannot be equalled. Shorter regimes of treatment with newer drugs, however, are almost certain to be used eventually.

The sanatorium will probably disappear as such. Beds occupied in 1972 were less than a quarter of those occupied in 1952. Already many such hospitals are providing care for non-tuberculous problems. Others have closed. Patients with infectious tuberculosis can usually be managed in a general hospital, given isolation facilities, but there will remain a small need for sanatorium-type care for specific groups, patients such as vagrants and alcoholics, when an admission of many months may need to be encouraged in order to supervise treatment and protect the community while curing the patient. The problem of the drug-resistant infection is very small and has diminished further with the availability of the newer drugs.

The use of BCG vaccination routinely has been re-evaluated recently and it is accepted that it is still a useful measure in the prevention of tuberculosis. Chemoprophylaxis in the strong tuberculin positive reactor, under the age of 5 years, even when there is no history of contact, is now widely practised and when there is a history of contact, a child or adolescent with a positive Heaf test should receive anti-tuberculosis treatment. For some time to come special expertise in the management of tuberculosis will be required but the chest clinics of the past will be incorporated into the general medical out-patient department with the possible temporary exception of the large urban clinics.

This leads to the future of the mass radiography service, which was so valuable in the past. Referral of symptomatic and high-risk patients yields more cases of active infection than mass screening, and the place of the latter was questioned many years ago. Radiological surveillance of high-risk groups, such as immigrants, diabetics and patients in institutions, hospital workers, and a number of others, rather than screening of the general population, should focus resources where they are most needed. Hopes of better results in treatment of lung cancer by early detection have been disappointing. This has led to the severe curtailment of the service: particularly the mobile part. Static units still function but they are likely to be phased out gradually. It goes without saying that there should be open access to radiological facilities in general hospitals for the GPs.

One of the most striking changes in the pattern of chest disease has been the dramatic increase in the incidence of lung cancer which has now reached epidemic proportions. The number of deaths in 1948 and 1968, respectively, from this disease were 10,379 and 29,045 (these figures include mediastinal, pleural, and lung tumours). Even allowing for the increase in population and its ageing, there has been an absolute increase in incidence. A tendency is now observable for the increase in deaths due to this cause to level off in younger males but the rise continues in females of all ages and in males over the age of 65. These facts can probably be explained on the basis of changes in smoking habits. Being a largely preventable disease it provides the challenge for the future. In the case of the other main smoking-related disease, chronic bronchitis, deaths from this in England and Wales have been fairly constant over a twenty-year period, 1947–67, with peaks occurring in years where there has been a hard winter, such as 1963. Working days lost through the disease causes a grave economic problem. The incidence of bronchitis, the largest cause of sickness absence from work could be halved if smoking were to cease. Unfortunately this greatest potential saving of life and benefit to health is unlikely to be achieved. Progress in the campaign against cigarette smoking is painfully slow. The reduction in smoking noted in 1971 following the report of the Royal College of Physicians, was not sustained beyond that year. Chest departments should be able to play a more active role here in the field of patient education and use of printed propaganda. Unfortunately the chest department is where the ravages of smoking are repaired with varying success. The real need is to prevent the habit, or in more realistic terms, to try and find a harmless substitute for it. There is a need for greater Government concern and tougher legislation, for example in the field of cigarette advertising.

Whether or not the levelling off in the incidence of lung cancer in the younger men continues, the need for thoracic surgical services will continue for the foreseeable future. Links with a thoracic centre should be close and a bronchoscopy service should be offered to all chest departments. Surgeons will always want to do their own bronchoscopies and these examinations by physicians should be rarely desirable, provided a good sputum cytology service, proved to be a remarkably accurate yet simple investigation, is available, particularly for the non-operable case. For these latter patients, access to a modern radiotherapy centre would be required.

Treatment of respiratory failure has been revolutionized by better understanding of its pathogenesis and the importance of controlled oxygen therapy. The introduction of a simple rebreathing method for measuring pCO_2 and the provision of a routine blood gas service from most hospital laboratories are remarkably recent developments of immense value. Chest physicians have properly become involved in intensive therapy units. These are commonly the responsibility of the anaesthetic departments, and chest physicians will vary in their wish to be closely involved routinely. In the case of respiratory failure, however, it is logical that they should be and furthermore that the physiotherapy department be intimately involved in the management of these patients. It is anticipated that these associations will grow. The appearance of the Vitalograph and the peak flow meter, both simple, compact, and robust instruments has contributed to the bringing of pulmonary physiological principles into clinical assessment, not only for the specialist but for any physician in an out-patient department. The quality of management of many respiratory problems depends increasingly on measurement of a number of basic pulmonary function tests, and evaluation of pulmonary function is becoming accepted outside specialist centres or even the largeı hospitals as important to the improved management of many chest diseases as a routine blood count in suspected anaemia. Expertise in basic pulmonary function assessment will be required in all chest physicians and simple laboratory facilities will have to be provided at district level. These provisions were envisaged by the Scadding report but not yet widely implemented. A pre-operative pulmonary assessment service would be a logical extension of these facilities.

Another major advance in the last ten to fifteen years has been the increased understanding of the nature of allergy, which has brought with it advances in the management of asthma. The marketing of disodium cromoglycate has proved not only an extremely valuable therapeutic advance but also has provided a research tool for further investigation of the disease. The mechanism by which organic dusts may produce allergic alveolitis has been intensively investigated and the list of implicated dusts grows still, helping to subdivide the pulmonary fibroses, already being scrutinized for associations with systemic disorders. Appreciation of the role of the aspergillus in asthma has also been a recent phenomenon and based on better understanding of its immunological associations. Asthma is likely to remain one of the major respiratory problems encountered in chest departments. Therapeutic advances are likely to continue as understanding of its mechanism grows. Familiarity with basic immunological principles will be essential to all chest physicians.

Industrial lung diseases continue to show a decline due to better dust control. Control of asbestos, the hazards of which have been known to some extent since the turn of the century, was slow to reach effectiveness but this has largely been remedied.

Unfortunately the neoplastic legacy from exposures up to forty years ago continues to be handed down to us.

Microbiology always played a vital role in the management of chest diseases and will continue to do so. Increased interest in virology is likely to continue.

In conclusion, contrary to predictions of fifteen to twenty years ago, the need for specialists in chest diseases has become unquestioned as the relative importance of non-tuberculous bronchopulmonary disease has grown. The many major advances in the understanding and treatment of many respiratory diseases has contributed towards making the specialty one of the most exciting to be involved in. The major goals—the eradication of tuberculosis, lung cancer and chronic bronchitis—may not sound practicable, but in theory could be easier to control than the common cold.

REFERENCES

HOSPITAL O AND M SERVICE REPORTS (3) (1959). *Chest Clinics* (London: HMSO).

CENTRAL HEALTH SERVICES COUNCIL STANDING TUBERCULOSIS ADVISORY COMMITTEE (1960). *The Future of the Chest Services* (London: HMSO).

—— (1968). *The Future of the Chest Services.* A Report by a Sub-Committee of the Standing Medical Advisory Committee (Chairman: J. C. Scadding) (London: HMSO).

RIDEHALGH, F. (1971). 'Medical staffing and training in chest diseases', *Br. med. J.* 1, 161–3.

ROYAL COLLEGE OF PHYSICIANS OF LONDON, COMMITTEE ON THORACIC MEDICINE (1971). *Report.* (London: RCP).

RESEARCH COMMITTEE OF THE BRITISH THORACIC AND TUBERCULOSIS ASSOCIATION (1971). 'A survey of tuberculosis mortality in England and Wales in 1968', *Tubercle*, 52, 1.

LEADING ARTICLE (1971). 'Preventable deaths', ibid., 52, 67.

SPRINGETT, V. H. (1971). 'Tuberculosis control in Britain 1945–1970–1995', ibid. 52, 136.

LEADING ARTICLE (1971). 'Fifty years of BCG', ibid. 52, 303.

LEADING ARTICLE (1972). 'Shorter treatment', ibid. 53, 265.

THE STANDING MEDICAL ADVISORY COMMITTEE FOR THE CENTRAL HEALTH SERVICES COUNCIL, THE SECRETARY OF STATE FOR SOCIAL SERVICES AND THE SECRETARY OF STATE FOR WALES (1973). *Tuberculosis: Epidemiology and Control* (London: DHSS).

GODBER, SIR GEORGE (1973). 'On the state of the public health', *Health Trends*, 5, 65.

Scottish Home and Health Department (1973). *The Future of the Chest Services in Scotland.* Report by a Sub-Committee of the Scottish Standing Medical Advisory Committee (Chairman: J. W. Crofton) (Edinburgh: HMSO).

Feinmann, L., and Martischnig, K. M. (1971). 'The decline and fall of the chest clinic', *Tubercle*, 54, no. 1, 77–82.

Some personal impressions of a move from Central London to the provinces

Part of my brief as a contributor to this collection of essays was to give some personal impressions of a move from Central London to the provinces. These are bound to be personal as I have no experience of training outside London or of a consultant appointment in London.

To be appointed to a consultant post alone is bound to lead to change. To take up an appointment outside Central London, having spent nearly ten years after qualification training entirely in London undergraduate and postgraduate teaching hospitals was bound to involve changes of major proportions. Looking back over fifteen months since my appointment in King's Lynn, most of the differences I encountered were predictable, few difficulties have been insurmountable, and many aspects of the move have given great pleasure.

In recent years more senior registrars have been looking outside London and other university towns for consultant posts as a first choice, rather than as last resort, when application to a teaching hospital has failed. Recent applicants for newly created posts in my own hospital have been very highly qualified indeed. Recent applicants for the GP and vocational training scheme here, which has enriched our junior staff, have been of remarkably high calibre, the sort of doctors who would rightly or wrongly in the past have been expected to pursue a hospital career. The reasons for this are well known to most of us. Links with London hospitals have enabled us to appoint good pre-registration house physicians and we have a steady trickle of medical students coming to us for their elective period or during holidays from all over the country.

The hospital, serving a rapidly expanding town, has increased its workload enormously in the past five years. In this time it has developed from a small, under-financed, relatively neglected hospital, to an extremely busy, lively district general hospital. With the creation of new consultant posts, skills have become available which had not existed before locally. In common with many other hospitals, space has been hard to find, huts and extensions have proliferated. The new DGH should have been half built by now, indeed many of the present staff were originally tempted here by the prospect of a new hospital and final approval of the building estimates are awaited with great anxiety.

It was astonishing to find such a rich variety of medical problems and a challenge to manage many, which had fallen within the practice of specialists only, before. This does have the corollary that specialist advice and some investigative facilities are often available only at a distance of forty to fifty miles at regional centres. Before sending a patient on such a journey it is necessary to be convinced of its necessity. In common with most district hospitals, regular out-patient clinics are run by our regional cardiologists and advice is always available from expert colleagues in neurology, neurosurgery, and cardiothoracic surgery in Cambridge and Norwich.

Having by far the highest number of patients per bed per year in the East Anglian Region, our in-patient medicine tends to be largely of emergency type and most investigation of patients is done in the out-patient department. The activities of a large geriatric department and the traditions of a large rural community to care for its elderly and infirm, means that patients are rarely in hospital for social reasons. The service commitment is therefore high and time has to be consciously made for teaching and postgraduate activities in order that it should not be swamped.

The increased interest of the colleges has helped to improve postgraduate training opportunities outside universities in those places where little existed before. Surveillance of training posts will continue to raise standards. In this region some individual enthusiasts have initiated MRCP teaching sessions to be held in turn in each interested centre. To find patients willing to take part in this is an easy task. A basic sciences course will be started next year.

Coming as a general physician with an interest in chest disease in place of a retiring pure chest physician has given limitless opportunities to follow a variety of interests and to develop the chest service in a new direction. The retreat into the general out-patient department, closure of several small outlying clinics and limitation of involvement with mass radiography, follows the national trend and has permitted a concentration of effort in the main department.

The creation of an additional general medical service to that already existing has been an absorbing task. As numbers of new patients have increased, very large numbers of old patients have been discharged to the care of their GPs. This has worked smoothly because of the high standard of general practice in the district. For the first time in my experience, a very close relationship exists between the GPs and the hospital, which makes continuity of care better for the patients and easier for us all.

Postgraduate activities have become livelier as a larger consultant staff has accumulated and more have been willing to take part in weekly clinicopathological conferences with a working lunch, and in evening lectures, which are increasingly well attended by all the local medical community. A completely new very well-equipped postgraduate centre will be completed in a month or so.

What therefore is missing? There is clearly less opportunity to attend open lectures and evening meetings in London because of the distance. Study leave, however, is encouraged and supported as at any teaching hospital and meetings of specialist societies tend to move round the country. A little more effort is needed to keep up with events and one must be prepared to travel. Many events of interest occur in the region itself and there is a well-trodden path from here to Cambridge. One thing particularly missed is a comprehensive library and in particular the inaccessibility in practical terms of the Royal Society of Medicine. A nucleus of journals and reference books does exist however and a willing librarian is able to obtain other publications within a very short time.

Opportunities for research are limited, partly due to lack of facilities and partly due to the heavy service load. This could be remedied to some extent in the future.

Aspects of work here which are more satisfying than in the capital are several. Some of these are associated with being appointed a consultant *per se*, but others do, I think, represent real differences. There is for example the strikingly greater variety and frequently florid nature of the medical problems. This is attributable at least partly to the large area served by the hospital and the phlegmatic character of many local patients. The out-patient department serves its true function in that many patients come already partly investigated and are known already to present difficult problems. One of the best aspects of coming here has been the scope for development of the job itself as opposed to taking over an established post. This must be an opportunity which rarely presents itself in a teaching hospital.

So far, all these impressions have concerned work alone, there are of course other facets of life in the provinces to be considered. Apart from economic factors driving young doctors out of London, there is the question of availability of particular facilities for recreation. This latter is a potent lure in Norfolk. A style of life belonging to what I regarded as a bygone era is still possible!

For me the move from London, which I still miss in some respects, has been a happy one. For others it clearly could not be. Teaching hospitals and district general hospitals are not strictly comparable and are not expected to provide the same facilities or postgraduate training. The modern district general hospital however, in some ways, provides the best of both worlds and will no doubt continue to attract more and more senior registrars even those with academic leanings or training in a specialty.

Services for the elderly

MICHAEL GREEN

S.F.—8

MICHAEL GREEN
MA, MB, MRCP
Consultant geriatrician

Services for the elderly

INTRODUCTION

Very many elderly people are mentally normal and physically fit. The adjective elderly can be dangerously misleading as it may be taken to mean that the person is an object of pity or suffers from senility—and there is no such disease anyway. As a group, however, chronologically old people often have serious problems of illness and disability, and with advancing age they have an increasing risk of medical and social breakdown at any time. The numbers and types of problems affecting the aged can cause great difficulties when planning and providing health care services. The demand for these services seems certain to increase during the next thirty years (1, 2).

Our aim should be to 'ensure attitudes and services that will allow old people to die at home, in comfort, and at an advanced age, having enjoyed their life up to the time of death' (3). This aim can only be achieved by providing effective and comprehensive services for practical and preventive health care. It requires more and better education for professional and voluntary workers in this field, and the middle-aged as well as the elderly. A greater priority must be given to allocating funds and resources to health and social services for the elderly, although more effective use of existing facilities is also needed.

By tackling the problems of old age in a positive way it should be possible to use limited money and manpower more effectively than at present. Positivity and optimism, however cautious, are also the best bases for finding out how best to practise medicine in old age, for proving that money needs to be spent to improve health and social circumstances, and for persuading more people to join in and help. Medical and social deficiencies are inextricably mixed in this situation, and a continuing injection of large sums of money is probably necessary to help correct existing deficiencies. This could provide for substantial and regular pension increases for the elderly, as well as for more staff, buildings, and equipment for health and social services. Inadequate income over ten or twenty years (for example, from retirement at 60 to ill health at 80) is probably an important factor in causing or precipitating medical and social deterioration.

The maintenance of good health and social wellbeing in the elderly is doubly justified. An effective, positive, and well-informed system of care in old age may not be much more costly in the long run than an ineffective, haphazard, and uncaring system. It would also reduce the burden of care on other people: there is about one frail elderly person for every six fit younger adults.

DEFINITION

Geriatrics, according to the Royal College of Physicians of London, is 'the branch of general medicine concerned with the clinical, preventive, remedial and social aspects of health and disease in the elderly' (1).

This has been described as a vague and unhelpful definition, but it must be remembered that two-thirds of the members of the College Committee were specialist physicians trying to encompass all aspects of medicine in old age.

Geriatrics is often described as an age-defined specialty, confined to the over-65s. The social, financial, and medical implications of retirement may be manifest within a very short space of time, but the average age of patients in most geriatric departments is in the 80s. This contrasts with other hospital departments where the average age in surgical wards may be 55–60, and about 60 in medical wards. It has also been suggested that as 'involutional' and degenerative disorders tend to start appearing in late middle age, geriatrics should start at 45! Prevention could include immediate or short-term measures to prevent breakdown in old age, or longer-term action starting in middle age aimed at reducing the incidence of diseases in elderly people.

The immediate and pragmatic approach to health and illness in old age is to use a team encompassing many disciplines, including doctors (hospital, specialist, family practitioner, and community physician), nurses, therapists, social workers, volunteers, and the elderly themselves. These people, gerontologists (who may also be 'practising' geriatricians), and other experts, should also be involved in the preventive approach. Both approaches require a realization that very few elderly people live in homes or hospitals, although many die in such institutions.

Any definition of geriatrics stands or falls by the effectiveness of our action to meet John F. Kennedy's requirement: 'It is not enough for a great nation to have added new years to life—our objective must also be to add new life to those years' (21 February 1963).

Past, present, future

It is convenient to discuss services for the elderly as if they were an ill patient, by using the problem-oriented medical records (POMR) approach (4). This is a particularly valuable tool in structuring, providing, and monitoring care for individual patients. Old people at home have an average of about six diagnoses (5), whilst geriatric in-patients have an average of more than eleven each, including social difficulties, laboratory abnormalities, and polypharmacy, as well as codable diagnoses. The multiplicity of factors affecting geriatric services, their interplay and modified presentation, and the difficulty in rendering them 'inactive', combine to enhance the value of the POMR approach. Only by identifying all problems and describing them as active or inactive (but with a potential for reactivation), can we begin to see which problems are curable and which irremediable. Insufficient money or personnel may make problems irremediable but at least they need to be clearly identified.

1. PAST HISTORY

A reduction in deaths in young and middle age, mainly from injury and infectious diseases, has led to a doubling of life expectation in the last 150 years. Women live longer than men, and there are many more elderly women. Rising age carries an increasing risk of multiple disease and disability, often irremediable, often mental as well as physical, and often inextricably mixed with social problems. These social problems are caused by inadequacies in provision, by the attitude of society to old people, and by a too humble outlook of old people themselves.

There is a great danger in retrospection in geriatrics, as the usefulness of past experience is limited. The problems of the past may have been superseded, and all that is left is praise of pioneering efforts. True pioneers would much rather see present knowledge and services as the springboard for the future, and not let geriatrics rest on the laurels of its first twenty-five years.

1.1. *Changes in disease and life expectation*

Large numbers of old people develop problems due to degenerative, vascular, neoplastic, and deficiency diseases. Old people are a new group of health resource users that did not exist at the beginning of the century. During this century, and accelerating in the last twenty-five years, spending on hospital and social services has increased many times, and taken an increasingly large slice of the health-spending cake. Not all old people necessarily need specialized geriatric attention, but the quality of their care is often reduced by the greater 'attractiveness' of other (younger) patient care groups, in a general setting or in specialized situations (for example, renal units, heart transplant research) in attracting money and people.

The image of geriatrics as unattractive has arisen partly because many diseases of old age are not apparently amenable to cure. Ischaemic heart disease, osteo-arthrosis, dementia, deafness, and incontinence are common problems, but a surprising amount can be done for old people who suffer from them. If improvement cannot be achieved then a positive decisive approach should benefit health services generally as well as the patient.

It is also possible that some of our present beliefs about health in old age are unproven or not entirely correct. If emotional conviction is not backed up with accurate observation, then wrong conclusions will follow, or intelligent planners will refute claims for more, and better services for the elderly. An example is the problem of hypothermia.

This is sometimes alleged to be the annual cause of hundreds of thousands of deaths in old people in the UK. Only about 100 deaths in over-65s are recorded on death certificates each year as being due to hypothermia. Between a quarter and three-quarters of a million over-65s are thought to have a deep body temperature of 35–35·5 °C at some time in the winter months. This is only a little higher than true hypothermia. The mortality of all diseases, except cancer, rises in the winter, but an accurate estimate of the true medical significance of hypothermia cannot be reached on the evidence available. Furthermore, this defect in our knowledge can be used by central and local planners as an excuse for not improving the thermal situation of old people by physical or financial means. Even if we were sure that lower-than-normal deep body temperatures were significantly morbid and mortal, the cost or effectiveness of preventive measures would still have to be established. Of course, there really is no excuse for any further delay in introducing ways of making old people warmer as a social benefit.

1.2. *Social structure*

The appearance this century of large cohorts of elderly people has altered the age-group proportions of the population. The over-65s have increased from one-twentieth to one-eighth of the population in seventy years. The actual increase in numbers is almost more important: there are now some seven and a half million over-65s in the UK. The care of ill and disabled old people has inevitably come to fall heavily on middle-aged and young people, as well as other old people.

It is interesting to speculate on the suggestion that we do not look after our old people as well as in other countries. There probably has been a true tendency for some families in the UK to look after aged relatives less satisfactorily than elsewhere, but the relatives of the 80- and 90-year olds will be middle-aged, often with children and commitments at work, and may be quite unable to cope physically and mentally. Some people who now survive into old age are very unfit, and their mental impairment and incontinence would strain the endurance of any devoted relatives or friends. The proportion and numbers of the over-65s really are much less in countries like India and China, where it is suggested that families always care for aged relatives. After all, about 95 per cent of our large elderly population are living out of hospitals and homes. Many are being cared for by devoted relatives, often single-handed.

Another point of speculation concerns the social attitudes of old people. Those who are old now were born in the Victorian era, and grew up through two world wars and major social, medical, technological, and geographical upheavals. The problems of caring for the old may change little in the next thirty to forty years, but the consumer voice may be much less retiring than at present, as those who are now middle-aged grow old.

1.3. *Health and social services*

Fourteen enthusiastic pioneers founded the Medical Society for the Care of the Elderly in 1948 (since renamed the British Geriatric Society). There are now almost 300 specialists in geriatric medicine in the UK, trying to improve and maintain the care of the elderly in most districts. There has been tremendous variation in the effectiveness with which the hospital-based geriatric service has really been able to establish its position as an important specialty in district general hospitals (DGHs), and forge effective links with GPs and community services. In spite of the size of geriatric departments, usually 100–300 in-patient beds, it has often been difficult to help care for all the elderly acute, medium-stay, and continuing care patients in each district's hospitals.

The proof that there should be such services comes from the benefit gained by people who have been rehabilitated, and by improved care for those who will never leave hospital. It is rare for either of these aims to be realized so well or so often by non-geriatric specialists (see also 2.7 and 4.4).

General practitioners have received most of their income from capitation fees for each person on their list. An increased fee for over-65s was introduced to acknowledge the need for more care for old people. It is often only regarded as payment for the number of calls made in response to specific demands, and not for preventive work. The demands of groups of old people, or difficult individuals, may be so great that a GP restricts his geriatric work (which he has the right to do).

The work of local authority and voluntary organizations, and their provisions for the elderly, have expanded greatly since 1948, although the National Assistance Act of that year still serves as the basis for many of the social services. This Act requested local authorities to provide homes for people in need of care or protection due to age, infirmity, or other reasons. There are several hundred beds in these homes in most districts. They have been complemented by services to support the aged in their own home and in sheltered accommodation.

The Local Authority Social Services Act of 1970 statutorily

obliged authorities to provide services for the elderly. The Seebohm reorganization which followed was intended to integrate services more efficiently, but the details of its implementation are still being sorted out. Local authority provisions, such as building more old peoples' homes, have always depended on raising revenue from local sources to add to central funding. It has often been inadequate to meet the tremendous cost of providing good personal services for the elderly, especially when more votes may be attracted by prestigious housing or educational developments.

Another piece of legislation which has failed in many respects to realize its promise is the Chronically Sick and Disabled Act, 1970. This was intended to improve the lot of handicapped people of all ages. Its recommendations covered the problems of physically and mentally handicapped persons and how they might be studied and solved (6). It embraced the work of health and welfare, education, traffic, and public building and housing authorities, but many of its most basic suggestions have not been acted on. How many public conveniences are convenient for even slightly disabled old people? The idea of information was central in the Act but a sad commentary on this is that only about one-eighth of handicapped people are registered as such, and three-quarters of the elderly who might be eligible for supplementary benefits did not know about their eligibility (7).

1.4. *Education*

There has been a serious lack of under- and postgraduate training in geriatric medicine, and of teaching for other health service personnel, volunteers, and the elderly. A very short paragraph about geriatric medicine is only just being included in the London University undergraduate curriculum. Only seven professorial units exist, four having been established in the last three years.

It is remarkable that such a large number of geriatric physicians has appeared when they have received little or no undergraduate exposure to even second-rate geriatrics. The number of specialists produced in the last twenty-five years is a tribute to the effectiveness of a few geriatric departments in converting some housemen and registrars to geriatrics, and of giving good senior registrar training. Other departments almost certainly deserve praise for teaching non-medical staff and volunteers, but many centres (of excellence?) of under- and postgraduate training, and the more ordinary service departments, can be criticized for not having produced teaching programmes for everybody in their district, including consultants and GPs.

1.5. *Changes in geriatrics*

The problems of starting geriatric services (and new departments are still being created) differ in some important ways from those of maintaining geriatric departments. It is helpful to analyse the changes in the work of a department established more than twenty years ago in west Cornwall (8).

In the early days much time was spent recruiting staff and getting patients out of bed. Now, more than twice as many patients are referred for admission, and many more ill patients are admitted, with an inevitable increase in the number of deaths. The local population has increased, the over-65s have increased considerably, and the mean age of admission has risen steadily. A drop in the proportion admitted of those referred is largely due to the establishment of more, and better, local authority services.

The English norm for planning geriatric beds is 10 per 1,000 over-65s. (Scotland works on a norm 50 per cent higher.) The West Country report states that they still have not realized the provision suggested in the lower norm, without even taking psycho-geriatric requirements into account. Planning norms are usually criticized, but in providing hospital and local authority services for the elderly they are often useless. More beds, and other facilities, are often required because of local factors. These include a higher-than-average elderly population, as in the southern 'Costa Geriatrica' and inner districts of cities, a scatter of beds with inadequate DGH facilities, and sometimes the difficulties inherent in rural areas where clinic, day-hospital, and day-centre attendance is difficult.

In any case these norms were established in 1954, the demand has changed since then, and there is a pressing need for updating the norms to provide more sophisticated and flexible ways of planning services.

1.6. *Psycho-geriatrics*

This is dealt with in detail by Dr C. Godber. The problems of the mentally infirm elderly have gradually been identified, and their needs categorized mainly on behavioural grounds (9). A basis for co-operation between psychiatrists and geriatricians (and psycho-geriatricians where they exist) has been developed in several places along the lines of a report from north-west London (10). Unfortunately psycho-geriatrics is an even later arrival in the resource market than geriatrics and psychiatry and is short of resources and staff. Dealing with the problems of elderly psychiatrically disturbed patients can be interesting and satisfying (11), but we must understand the outsider's view of the specialty as the custodial care of confused and incontinent old ladies.

1.7. *Attitudes*

Many of the historical reasons for the wrong and obstructive attitudes about good, positive care for the elderly have already been touched on. These reasons are often the cause of the existing deficiencies in geriatric provision (12) which are perpetuated by a vicious circle of defective education about old age, sometimes leading to mismanagement and even neglect.

An awareness of the possibilities of good management of old people is often sadly lacking in senior people in the health service. Awareness might have the benefit of improving their own medical work and the prospects for their own and their relatives' old age. Faulty attitudes in dealing with specific management problems will be dealt with later, but a recent survey (13) has highlighted how teaching hospital consultants can alter the general attitudes of junior doctors for the worse. Senior medical students had liked geriatrics and were patient/treatment orientated, but junior hospital medical staff had a less favourable attitude and were education/career orientated. The change of attitudes must surely be blamed on attitudes the junior doctors encountered after qualifying.

1.8. *Past into present*

As Townsend says: 'The treatment in particular of many of the aged, chronic sick and disabled, mentally ill and mentally handicapped, remains scandalously poor and can in the long run be dramatically improved only by a redefinition of health and health needs, and by a reconstruction of professional values and organization, the education and involvement of the patient, and the establishment of social equality' (14).

2. THE PRESENT

The principles of geriatrics are well established and are applicable to old people in and out of hospital, in health and illness. Old age should not exclude a patient from the best care possible. Care can mean alleviation or positive management of chronic and terminal disease. As we cannot ensure good health into a happy old age for everybody, the quality of life should be maintained as long as possible. The objectives have been described as 'disease control and the maintenance of life of optimum quality in as many elderly as possible' (15).

2.1 *Diagnosis and positive management*

Major functional changes tend to occur in the elderly: pain, sensation, balance, temperature control, and thirst are all impaired. These are pathophysiological changes and are usually due to the disease processes mentioned in 1.1. The first step in managing the elderly is the ascertainment of ill health, by accurate identification of these diseases and of disordered bodily function (16).

Identifying and treating physical, mental, and social disorders should lead to action to alleviate if possible, but certainly to prevent further deterioration. An understanding of the pathology of disease processes, and of the importance of social and financial factors should also lead to effective prophylactic measures.

Accurate diagnosis is the keystone. For instance, no-one is senile, incontinence is due to something (a catheter treats a symptom not a diagnosis), mental confusion can be caused by depression, delirium, or dementia, sometimes in the same person, and two of these can be cured. Anything can happen in old age (except pregnancy), but common things are common and are often incurable. Multiple pathology and modified presentation conspire to confuse the diagnostician; one symptom can be caused by severe disorders (for example, constipation due to years of over-purgation, depression, hypothyroidism, and codeine given for arthritis) or one disorder can have several causes (for example, iron-deficiency anaemia from poor diet, malabsorption, and blood loss). There is a danger that over-zealous diagnosis may lead blindly to treatment and harm or kill. Even when we are aware of the dangers of polypharmacy it is impossible to avoid more than half our in-patients regularly receiving three or more drugs.

These simple remarks about diagnosis and management are necessary, as inadequate examination and diagnosis, and careless, uninformed prescribing are still all too common in old age.

2.2. *Hospital services*

Geriatric services can be marvellous, admired by patients and respected by colleagues. Sadly, there are serious defects in all parts of the country with geriatric patients badly housed, low nurse/patient ratios, and grossly inadequate medical staff (12). The Hospital Advisory Service has constantly reiterated the defects it has encountered, and pointed out the continuing inertia and even positive antagonism of many teachers and specialists in other fields. It has commented on the disparity between creed and practice even in geriatric units; in one of its reports the problem of pressure sores gets one and a half pages including comments like 'more than half the ripple beds were not working' (17).

The ideal minimum provision of 120-bed geriatric departments, at least half the beds at the DGH and a numerically adequate staffing establishment, is still a pipe dream in many districts. At present each geriatrician on average serves 250,000 people, has almost 300 in-patients, admits 800 people annually, and deals with more than 100 GPs. Although geriatricians are directly responsible for only two-fifths of the hospital beds occupied by the elderly, and less than one-fifth of elderly people admitted to hospital, their patients are usually much more disabled than elderly people in general wards. (Figures [18] derived mainly from a paper [19] given at a DHSS/British Geriatric Society Conference.)

It is possible to achieve a remarkable turnover in geriatric beds. Death, or early discharge of many patients, were the only ways of achieving an annual admission rate of 1,800 people into a 250-bed geriatric unit including an annexe of 70 continuing-care beds. The trouble is that this sort of 'performance' and restoration of independence in many old people can justifiably be criticized if the geriatrician is not also prepared to *help* in organizing the care of chronically disabled old people. Doctors and nurses in other departments often complain of blocked beds when they see disabled elderly people requiring little 'active' treatment remaining in their beds. More than a tenth of patients admitted to medical wards stay more than thirty days, the majority are elderly women, and many have had a stroke (20, 21). There is considerable scope for improving the outlook for such patients by liaison between geriatric and general medical departments (4.3), by getting rehabilitation going immediately and by active investigation of the avenues of possible discharge, to home, homes, and community hospitals. This can all be done without necessarily transferring the patient to geriatric wards; such transfer can be for further rehabilitation or for continuing long-term care. One-fifth of geriatric patients are stroke patients (21), and strokes and other disorders of locomotor, central nervous, and cardiac systems account for many of the continuing-care patients remaining in hospital for the rest of their lives.

It is a remarkable situation, akin to psychiatry, that geriatricians take over the care of a large number of patients from other doctors. These other doctors often react antagonistically to these elderly patients and feel that they are stopping them doing their proper work which 'should be more acute and effective from the patient's point of view and interesting from the point of view of the doctor' (22). A questionnaire was circulated prior to my present appointment to all the other consultants (in a teaching hospital). There had been no specialized geriatric service or teaching previously. The majority thought that an important function of geriatric departments was to transfer patients from their beds. A senior physician even asked whether geriatricians admit cases. Even if a geriatrician is prepared to take a substantial number of his admissions by transfer from other wards and is prepared to allocate a major proportion of his beds to permanently disabled old people, there may still be insufficient 'long-stay' beds to take all such patients from the community and away from the wards where they were originally admitted.

Some longer-stay patients are ostensibly waiting for admission to a home, but remain in hospital indefinitely because they are almost too frail to be coped with out of hospital. Some are 'acceptable' but remain in hospital because, as a result of competition from old people in crisis in the community, they are low on the priority list. Others are too frail for existing sheltered accommodation or homes to cope with: surprisingly a few of these return to their own home, if they have one, although it may cost relatives, friends, and supporting services very dear. The most difficult problem in this long-term hospital-community care situation is how best to cope with the elderly mentally infirm, particularly those with dementia. When physical problems dominate the situation medical or geriatric in-patient care seems logical. The confused, sometimes incontinent, often highly mobile, old lady who has recovered from the reason for admission, and may not necessarily have deteriorated very much from her previously impaired mental state, is often very difficult to get home, or into a home, or into a psychiatric ward.

2.3. *General practitioners*

About 95 per cent of old people are not in hospital, and GPs provide their primary medical care. The fact of having large numbers of elderly people to deal with does not guarantee expertise. Many GPs have not had any specific under- or post-graduate training in geriatrics, although postgraduate meetings on geriatric topics are increasingly popular.

The GP tends to come into contact with ill old people, often living alone, and unhappy. 'Monitoring demand gives a false impression of actual medical need' in old age, and general practice is 'inadequate to deal with elderly patients who for a variety of reasons do not report their illnesses until they present as geriatric tragedies or social upheaval' (23). Thus, a GP providing an immediate service in times of crisis should also be trying to develop a preventive approach.

All too often general practice may still be a rather haphazard day-to-day business with immediate and long-term care of the elderly a low priority. This is particularly true of large towns and cities where the picture may be one of ageing, single-handed practitioners, who often qualified in other countries, working in poor premises and being bypassed by advances in medical care (24). These strictures imply that effective GP–geriatric service liaison in large conurbations is likely to be tenuously ephemeral or nonexistent. General practitioners, however, are not entirely to blame. Many of the crises and strains producing this situation are caused by defects in hospital services, local authority provision and the relative poverty of so many of Britain's pensioners. The GP is in an important central position and may not only provide a poor medical service for pensioners on his list, but also pessimistically perpetuate adverse assumptions about the inevitability and irreversibility of the problems of old age.

Some GPs, whether single-handed or working in groups, are providing a very good service. One important way they have managed this is by sharing some of the problems of their aged clients with other people. The community (district nurse), health visitor (perhaps specializing as a geriatric visitor), and social worker can work in this way to help with, or prevent problems (4.4).

2.4. *Community health and social services*

The 1974 Reorganization Act envisages better integration of health and social services for the elderly through the broad scope of district management teams, joint liaison committees, and community health councils, and through the specific work of health care planning teams (HCPT). Unfortunately the continuing dichotomy of health and social services in their funding and machinery for action, will probably perpetuate many of the current problems in providing services for the elderly. The tremendous goodwill to make the integrated approach work may all too easily be dissipated by there being too little money to pay for personal supporting services (for example home helps, meals-on-wheels, day and night nursing, day-centres and clubs, laundry facilities) and for sheltered and residential accommodation. There needs to be a tremendous speeding up of such simple things as getting alterations in disabled peoples' homes.

Newly created community physicians (CPs) will be responsible for each district, and some may have a special interest in the care of the elderly but, however well CPs pinpoint the needs of the elderly and supply the HCPTs with local and national information, the implementation of HCPT recommendations will almost certainly demand the spending of more money as well as improving the efficiency of existing resources.

It is surprising how much of its revenue the DHSS spends on benefits for young and middle-aged working people and their families rather than on health at all ages and social services for the aged. Social service departments all too often have to compete against more powerful voices in the national and local sector for funds for all their work, and in particular may fail to provide comprehensive resources for the elderly. This is particularly anomalous when their work often overlaps with other, better-funded departments such as housing and education.

There has been, however, a steady expansion of the social work department, and of specialized services. These include supporting services to maintain an independent existence at home, sheltered accommodation and residential homes, as well as pre-retirement courses and leisure activities for the aged. In all these spheres local and national voluntary organizations have been invaluable assistants, and have even performed much-needed research and publicity (see *Age Concern Today* [25]). These organizations have helped to identify many of the problems of the elderly in the community and tried to get rid of them. Age Concern has always emphasized the problems of the shortage of money for pensions and funding services for the elderly, and the need to improve these will almost certainly be a feature of the 'Manifesto' for old age they are preparing to submit to the Government.

As in 2.2, the postscript to this section must be a mention of the elderly mentally infirm. Supporting and residential services fall far short of the need. Only about 15 per cent of demented elderly people are in institutions, and community services are still uncertain how best to help them. Even when local authorities have some residential accommodation for them (and only a tiny number have), it has been provided without knowing whether it is best to have homes only for demented old people, or whether they should be mixed with the more normal welfare home resident (26).

2.5. *Staffing*

Inadequate teaching curricula, antagonistic attitudes in other specialties, and the deficiencies in geriatric services have been blamed for the difficulties of staffing geriatric departments. Subsidiary reasons have included lack of financial reward due to the virtual absence of private practice, and the low incidence of merit awards. More than four-fifths of geriatric consultants have whole-time contracts, compared with only one-quarter of those in general medicine. Expansion of all grades in the geriatric establishment has been so rapid since 1948 that it is not surprising that there are many vacancies, especially as the majority of entrants into the geriatric job lists are after-qualification converts. I am indebted to Dr A. M. S. Mason of the Medical Manpower Division of the DHSS for the graphs and information used as the basis for discussing geriatric staffing problems. The graphs are virtually self-explanatory and the brief comments are my opinions, not his.

Fig. 1 shows that geriatric consultants' bed-loads have decreased over the years, but are still ridiculously high, especially as occupancy is well over 90 per cent. As the number of consultants has risen the annual workload (judged by deaths and discharges) has dropped.

Figs. 2, 3*a* and *b*, 4*a* and *b*, and 5*a* and *b* show the posts available and filled, and the post-holders' country of origin, for senior hospital officers (SHOs), registrars, senior registrars, and consultants in geriatrics. There are no figures for unfilled SHO posts. Table 1 compares the posts details of successful candidates, and details of previous appointments of new consultants in geriatrics and general medicine.

TABLE 1

New consultants, March 1970 to November 1973: geriatrics and general medicine

A. DETAILS OF POSTS REVIEWED		
Details	*Geriatrics*	*General medicine*
Period reviewed	March 1970– November 1973	January 1970– April 1973
Number of posts reviewed	118	116
Posts filled (%)	64	96
Average number candidates per post	4·2	8·2

B. DETAILS OF THE SUCCESSFUL CANDIDATES: 75 (GERIATRICS) AND 116 (GENERAL MEDICINE)		
Characteristics	*Geriatrics*	*General medicine*
Trained in England (%)	55	86
Male (%)	90	93
Average age (years)	39·9	36·6
Average time SR (years)	1·8	3·5

C. DETAILS OF THE PREVIOUS APPOINTMENT OF SUCCESSFUL CANDIDATES		
Previous post	*New consultants (%)*	
	Geriatrics	*General medicine*
Consultant	16	7
Locum consultant	11	2
SHMO/MA	8	2
SR	64	85
Academic/research	0	3
Other	1	1

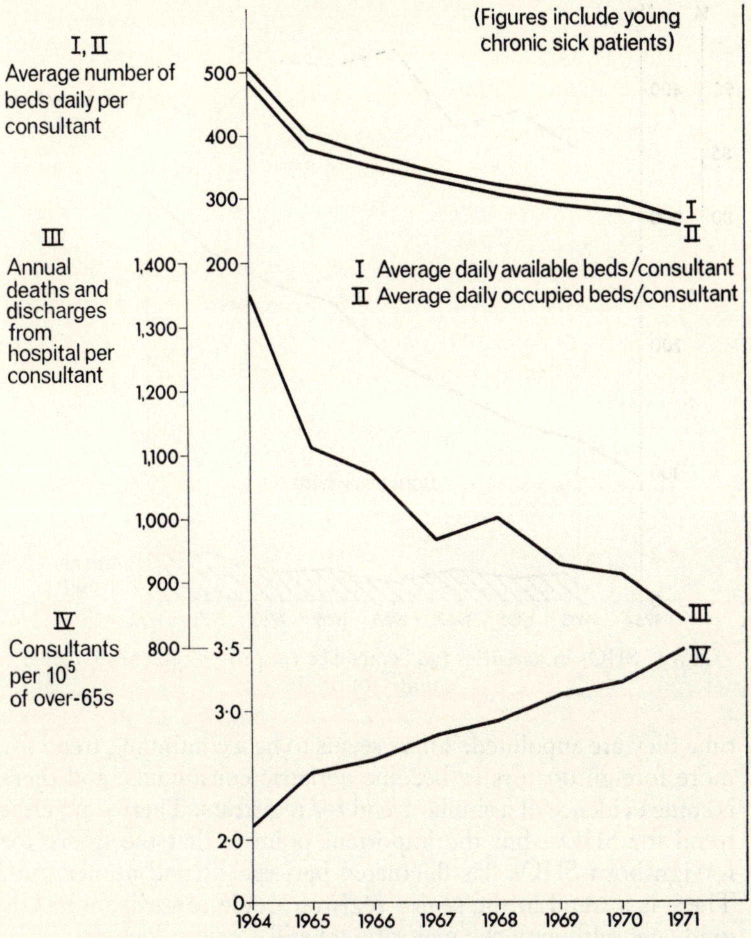

FIG. 1. Consultants in geriatrics: 'workload' (1964–71).

About 30 per cent of senior registrar, 15 per cent of consultant, and 10 per cent of registrar posts were unfilled on 30 September 1972. These unfilled vacancies seemed to represent a worsening trend to more vacancies in the two senior grades. Almost 90 per cent of SHOs, 85 per cent of registrars, and 25 per cent of consultants had been born abroad. My impression is that the majority of geriatric consultants born (not necessarily qualified) abroad have, or are in the process of obtaining, British nationality by the

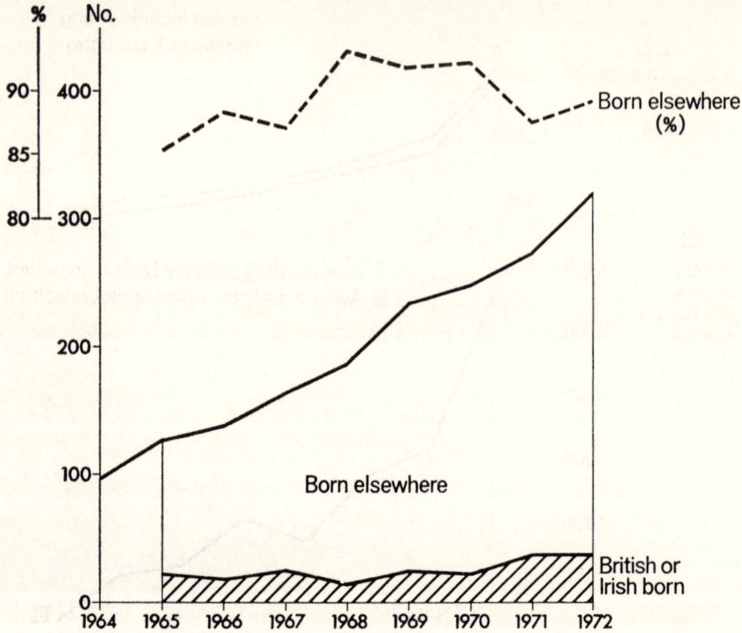

FIG. 2. SHOs in geriatrics (30 September 1964 to 30 September 1972): country of origin.

time they are appointed. There seems to be a continuing trend for more foreign doctors to become geriatric consultants, and there is some evidence of a similar trend for registrars. There is no clear trend for SHOs, but the important point is that the figure for foreign-born SHOs has fluctuated between 85 and 95 per cent. There is a trend in the senior registrar grade towards more UK graduates, although the majority are still foreign doctors.

Most senior registrars and consultants ought to have had considerable training in geriatrics and possess higher qualifications. The over-all quality of geriatric consultants is sometimes questioned on the grounds that many were appointed too young and/or with insufficient general or senior registrar training. Table 1 confirms the shortness of senior registrar experience in recently appointed consultants, but also reveals that the average age of appointment was almost 40 years, and older than in general medicine. This is probably due to the wide variety of careers that have preceded geriatric senior registrar and consultant appointments (general practice, other medical specialties, services, research, work abroad) as well as 'organized' vocational training leading directly into a geriatric career.

Foreign graduates have been a vital factor in the staffing of our geriatric services, as in other fields, including general practice. Almost 2,000 overseas doctors were given full registration in 1973, about 350 were granted provisional registration and well over 2,000 were granted temporary registration for the first time. Many of these doctors took junior geriatric posts. These doctors may have had no undergraduate geriatric teaching (but remember our deficiencies), and come from countries where life expectation is shorter and social attitudes different, but possibly more sympathetic to the elderly. These factors and language problems may make it difficult for foreign doctors in SHO grades, but should not affect those in higher posts.

The General Medical Council is proposing to start a simple examination of language and clinical competence next year, to be operated in parallel with an improved clinical attachment assessment scheme. This will only be a test of overseas doctors wishing to work in the hospital service under temporary registration. This examination could reduce the number of foreign doctors available to us. About 4,500 foreign doctors came to the UK and 1,500 had clinical attachments in 1973. We do not want non-English-speaking, poorly trained, or incompetent doctors, but exclusion by such an examination is not as simple an issue as it may seem. Only just over 90 per cent of English, and just under 90 per cent of Scottish, entrants pass the US Educational Council for Foreign Medical Graduates entrance examination (ECFMG), and these are doctors already qualified in the UK. The problem of relying on foreign doctors is particularly critical as there is a net loss of the order of 300 British graduates annually. This is a substantial loss as our annual output of medical graduates is only around 3,000. A reduction in the number of foreign graduates coming into geriatrics, and a continued loss of British graduates in all fields may rapidly reverse the slightly more optimistic geriatric recruitment figures for the period since 1972, when the statistics used in the graphs were produced.

The implementation of more socially organized medical care is expected in the USA in the next few years. This will almost certainly lead to an increase in the number of doctors required to

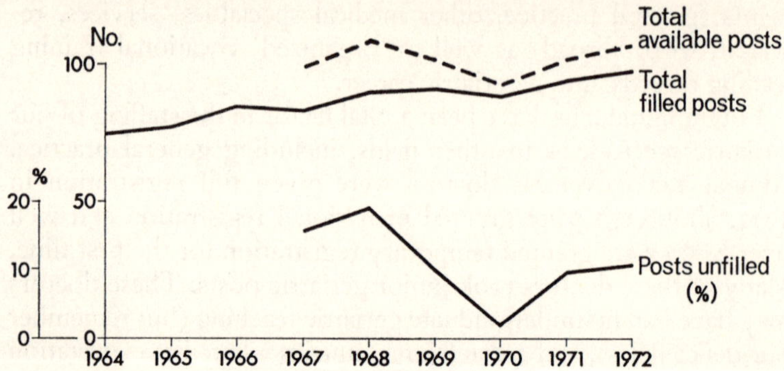

FIG. 3*a*. Registrars in geriatrics (30 September 1964 to 30 September 1972): posts available and posts filled.

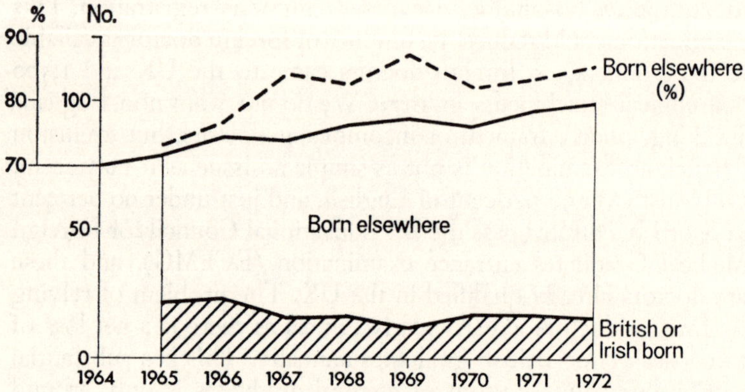

FIG. 3*b*. Registrars in geriatrics (30 September 1964 to 30 September 1972): country of origin.

run their system and a further net loss of British and foreign graduates. There have been some restrictions on medical graduates leaving 'backward' countries but a fair number still manage to leave. Any increase in the restrictions stopping this flow of doctors would tend to reduce the number of potential British immigrants still further.

It is worrying to note that only two-thirds of the advertised geriatric consultant posts were filled from March 1970 to November 1973 (Table 1). There were half the candidates for geriatrics that there were for general medicine, and successful candidates in geriatrics had come from a variety of previous posts, whereas nearly all the general medicine consultants came straight from senior registrar appointments. This is not necessarily a bad thing for geriatrics, although on average, those who had been senior registrars had only spent half as long in post. Vacating consultant and locum consultant jobs to become a consultant elsewhere is also a feature of geriatric promotion, and may be rewarding for the successful candidate but very disturbing to the departments they leave.

The ratio of consultants to senior registrars has fallen steadily over the years to the present ratio of about one senior registrar to every five consultants. The expansion of the senior registrar grade in geriatrics seems sometimes to have been to provide a pair of hands, which might have been better provided by a registrar. New registrar posts have been created in geriatrics, but few registrar posts have been established by the redeployment of 'unnecessary' jobs in other fields. The hope that availability of posts in good departments would attract doctors into geriatrics has apparently not been realized.

It is also interesting to note the number of women doctors working in geriatrics: 7 per cent of consultants, 25 per cent of senior registrars, 10 per cent of registrars, and about 25 per cent of SHOs. This suggests that we might be tapping a useful pool of doctors and that the number of women geriatric consultants could rise in the future.

Perhaps the most worrying features of Dr Mason's and other DHSS statistics (27) are the number of posts unfilled, and the number vacant for at least six months. There were 180 posts of all grades unfilled in 1970. Thirty-three consultant posts were vacant for at least six months in 1972, and the total number of

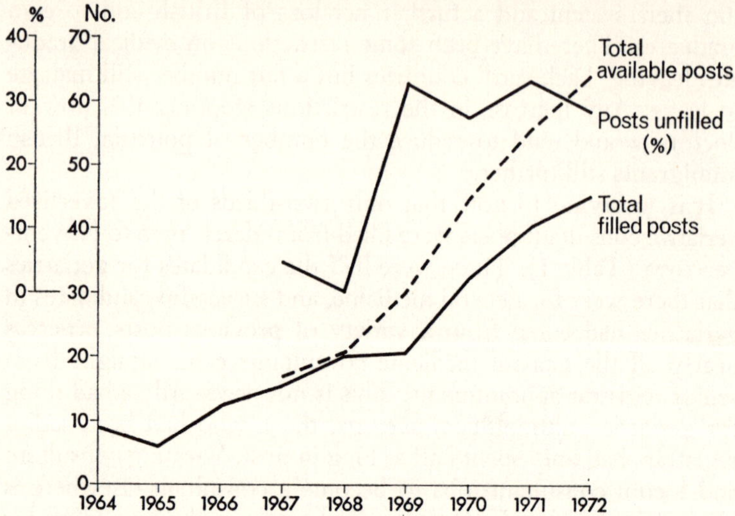

FIG. 4*a*. Senior registrars in geriatrics (30 September 1964 to 30 September 1972): posts available and posts filled.

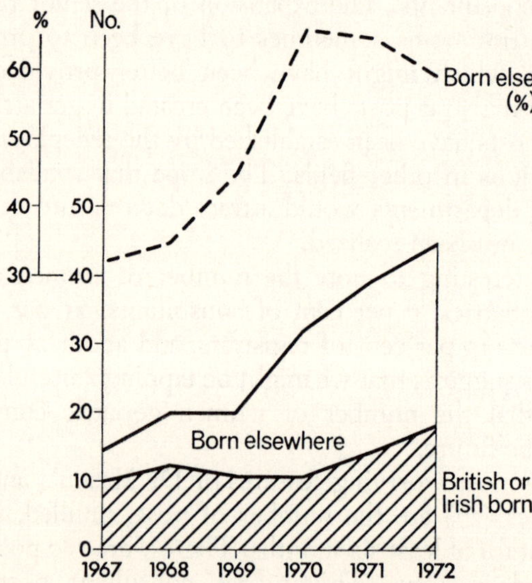

FIG. 4*b*. Senior registrars in geriatrics (30 September 1964 to 30 September 1972): country of origin.

consultants in post on 30 September 1972 was 246 (236 whole-time equivalents). A British Geriatrics Society memorandum has commented (28) that some members even questioned 'the survival of the specialty in its present form', because of the recruitment problem. Of course many specialties have a large number of unfilled posts; a total of 1,000 unfilled consultant posts in the UK is often quoted. This is almost certainly an overestimate, and includes posts in the process of being filled and others which are virtually non-viable because there are only two or three sessions. The apparently worrying number of unfilled posts in geriatrics is therefore only part of the spectrum of difficulties in filling consultant posts generally.[1]

It is often alleged that major reasons for potential geriatricians being discouraged are the poor quality of junior medical staff, and the difficulty of getting a reasonable staffing establishment and of filling it. The figures available do not really allow one to comment on these points, as they do not reveal the quality of the staff, nor indicate whether individual departments that do have inadequate establishments also have the greatest difficulty in getting staff. This may be true, but it could be just another example of a damaging misconception.

2.6. *Money*

The hope that the reorganized Health Service will improve the integration and performance of hospital–GP–community care resources for the elderly may founder on the lack of money allocated for this sector of care. We are devoting a smaller, and diminishing proportion of our total monetary resources to health services than many other advanced industrial societies, including most of the EEC countries (14). There is also disproportionate

1. The manpower figures on 30 September 1973 were similar to those discussed: about 26 per cent of senior registrars, 11 per cent of consultants, and 8 per cent of registrar posts were unfilled; almost 90 per cent of SHOs, 85 per cent of registrars, and 32 per cent of consultants had been born abroad; 8 per cent of consultants, 13 per cent of senior registrars, 10 per cent of registrars, and about 20 per cent of SHOs were women; there were 96 posts of all grades unfilled, 32 consultant posts had been vacant for at least six months, the total number of consultants in post was 271 (262 whole-time equivalents). Additional information is now available that very few women doctors have returned to geriatrics in a part-time capacity.

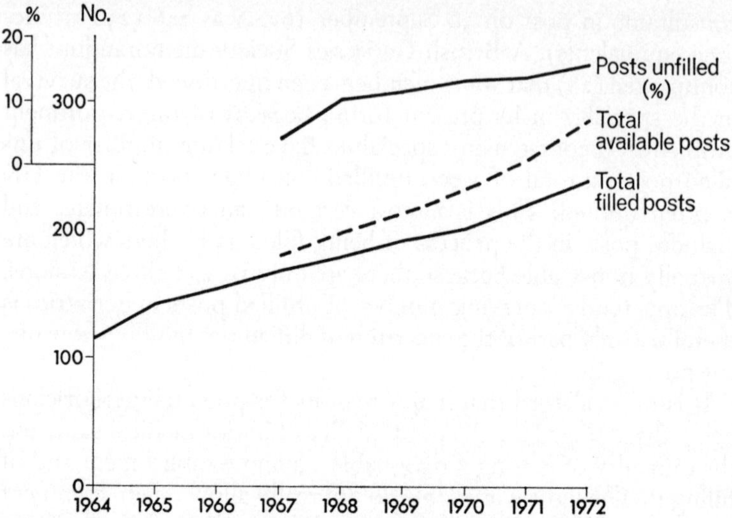

FIG. 5*a*. Consultants in geriatrics (30 September 1964 to 30 September 1972): posts available and posts filled.

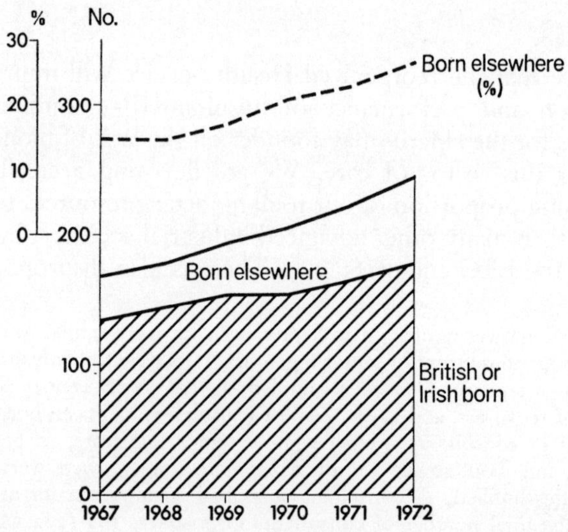

FIG. 5*b*. Consultants in geriatrics (30 September 1967 to 30 September 1972): country of origin.

spending of this amount of money, as we respond to 'the demands, not the needs' (29) when apportioning government and local spending. Even after more than twenty-five years of an organized NHS, and the apparent partial success of providing specialized geriatric services, the aged, the poor, and those in lower social classes still have high morbidity/mortality rates, often unchanged for decades. Other inequalities are demonstrated by the lower costs of personal services (food, laundry, heating) for the elderly in their 'non-acute' hospitals, compared with the 'acute' hospitals. The lower cost of some of the staffing and equipment does not entirely account for the discrepancies and could be signs of inadequate resource allocation. Elderly patients may be smaller than younger patients and 'need' less calories, but the food they should have may be more expensive, and the costs of laundry and heating should be higher in old age if the needs are really being met. In other words, services for the elderly are really rather ineffective (have not improved the natural history of diseases enough) and inefficient (have not used people and materials well) (30), largely as a result of inadequate finance.

Britain's extremely low health expenditure is not only 'a measure of more economical delivery of centrally financed services' (29), but a measure of insufficient total and disproportionate spending. There is disproportionate spending: Scotland is better off than England and Wales (generally and for geriatrics), and south-eastern England is better off than the north-east or Midlands; Sheffield often comes at the bottom of many of the analyses of resource provision.

Spending on local authority services is also too low as a result of inadequate central funding, and local difficulties in obtaining adequate rate apportionment for social services spending. These problems come to a head in areas like the south coast, where the over-65 population in some towns is more than 35 per cent of the total. Most of these towns have a geriatric bed allocation well below the planning norm (31).

Another financial 'trap' adds to the monetary inadequacies of health and social services for pensioners. Most of our people are rather poor, do not have large savings, and many rely on State pensions for their main income. The interactions of three factors conspire to produce a poverty trap after retirement (32):

(*a*) Extra pension rights can be earned to augment the State pension (by occupational schemes, State graduated pensions, or by working on for up to five years after retirement).

(*b*) These and supplementary benefits and rent and rate rebates available to supplement the basic State pension are means-tested.

(*c*) Part-time work after retirement may cause loss of the right to any supplementary benefits, and eventually to the loss of any of the State pension. Extra earnings could also provoke heavy income tax liabilities.

The effect of these three factors is to suppress many pensioners' income below the poverty line, and they cannot get any higher. The majority of those eligible for supplementary benefits do not know about or do not claim them; about a million old people are in this category!

Inadequate pensions may not only lead to ill-health, but are likely to reduce the quality of life every week the pensioner is drawing them. Services for the elderly should not be seen as just trying, rather ineffectively, to cope for ill old people in hospital and frail old people in homes or their own home, but also as helping provide comfort, happiness and independence.

After all, it is a Department of Health and *Social Security*.

2.7. *Geriatrics versus general medicine*

This should be an unnecessary section as geriatrics is part of general medicine, is general medicine in old age, and virtually anything medical can happen in old people. The combined effect of defective education (1.4), wrong attitudes (1.7), and staffing difficulties (2.6) all conspire to make this a controversial and topical subject.

The first priority is to confirm that geriatrics has a right to its present position as a separate specialty in the general field of medicine. The approach of many non-geriatric physicians is 'organ-oriented' but the geriatric patient must be considered as a whole. Elderly patients usually have many medical things wrong with them in addition to social disability, and it would be quite impractical to call in several specialists to see every aged person in hospital. The need for accurate diagnosis in old age has already been stressed, and where necessary specialists can help to elucidate diagnoses or advise on management. Geriatric physicians use the diagnostic information from history, examination, and investigations, including social work, occupational and physiotherapy assessment, to diagnose functional ability and potential.

The special skills of nurses and other therapists in geriatric departments and the provision of properly designed chairs, beds, and other equipment help to continue this functional approach. The special skills include awareness of mundane facts often lost sight of in general wards. Many old people are in hospital for the first time and can so easily become confused, especially if they have some deterioration of hearing or sight which aggravates the disorientation caused by removal from familiar surroundings. Immobilization, by confining them to bed or chair, possibly heightened by locomotor disease (stroke, arthritis) and sedatives may increase confusion and produce incontinence and pressure sores. The geriatric team will all be aware of how common mental impairment is in elderly patients even when admission policies exclude psycho-geriatric cases. A study of unselected geriatric admissions showed that only half were mentally normal (33). Ten per cent were depressed, 10 per cent confused, and 30 per cent demented.

Another major feature of the inexperience of generalists in dealing with elderly patients is in their prognostications. It has been shown that the prognosis was wrong in nine-tenths of patients transferred to a geriatric unit (34). Almost a third of the transferred patients were discharged and only 10 per cent lived more than ten months and could really be classed as long-stay. Faulty prognosis in most cases errs on the side of pessimism, many physicians believing that many old patients will never recover sufficient function after a stroke or that it is quite impossible for an old lady to live alone again.

The generalist or non-geriatric specialist rarely develops a positive diagnostic approach to the elderly to identify and assess physical, mental, functional, and prognostic features. He may also find it difficult to know when to investigate in depth and to treat energetically and when not to.

In particular, the management of death in old age still needs a positive and caring approach (35) so often lacking in general wards. Something like one-half of all deaths are in non-psychiatric hospitals; the majority of these deaths are in old people and one-third of patients admitted to geriatric departments die there.

These departments must therefore have good equipment and amenities for dying patients to complement the skilled terminal care of a geriatric team. This is rarely possible in general wards where the management of death in old age is often haphazardly organized by junior staff in the corner of a ward.

The geriatrician is much more involved with the hospital–GP–social service community approach to old people than is the general physician. He often sees ill old people in their own homes and may do several domiciliary visits a week. Out-patient clinics and day-hospitals (36) also serve as further links with the community to maintain old people out of hospital. There are well over a hundred geriatric day-hospitals in the country now. They are used mainly to prevent unnecessary admission, to hasten discharge, and sometimes just to maintain physically and mentally disabled old people at a reasonable level of functional ability indefinitely. Other practices linking hospital and community care are schemes for six weeks in and six weeks out (37), holiday admissions (38), and a five-day rehabilitation ward (39). There is a danger that these various arrangements utilize hospital services for people who could be cared for elsewhere but they do exemplify services not in the general physicians' orbit. A review of other past and present developments in geriatrics (19) also mentions the important research work done by geriatric departments working in and out of hospitals. Other important developments have come from specialist groups such as the British Geriatrics Society, the British Society for Research on Ageing, and the British Society for Social and Behavioural Gerontology and from broader-based groups such as Age Concern and the Geriatric Care Association.

Only two-fifths of the over-65s in hospital are in geriatric beds and geriatricians deal with less than one-fifth of over-65s admitted to hospital (19). The greater age and dependency of the geriatric patients has been mentioned. Good geriatricians do expect to advise on the care of old people in colleagues' wards as well as helping by transferring some of them. An analogy can be made with diabetes mellitus: many diabetics will be admitted under the care of the diabetic specialist, many into other wards. Some of those in other wards will benefit by specialist diabetic advice and some will need transfer to his care. All diabetics coming to the hospital should benefit by the teaching and research work of the diabetic department.

It has been proposed that a good solution to the shortage of geriatricians, and to the divergences of opinion between general and geriatric physicians, would be to appoint more general physicians with an interest in geriatrics. This would need a good existing geriatric service in the district if it was to work at all, but these appointments are often proposed as an alternative to full geriatric posts, not to complement them. These combination doctors often opt for the next vacant fully general job and one wonders how much energy they have devoted to their geriatric work.

A broadly acceptable referral and admission policy for geriatric patients has been described (15). It is based on specific age cut-offs and on an admission and follow-up policy based on whether the elderly patient has single system or multisystem involvement and on the degree of disability. It is an individual view, and its wider implementation would depend on the local facilities as well as the attitudes of the other physicians. It is a brave attempt to show how friction between hospital colleagues, GPs, and geriatric departments can be minimized by a sensible and organized approach; it is realized after a fashion in some of our best geriatric departments.

The relevance of this detailed discussion of the misunderstandings between geriatricians and general physicians and of the special features of geriatrics can be demonstrated by quoting from some recent correspondence. This followed a leading article in *The Lancet* that stated: 'The realities demand reappraisal of our attitudes. Geriatrics is medicine and may be the general medicine of the future' (40). A general physician commenting on this summarized many of the important points of geriatric medicine but said that geriatric physicians must help shovel away the non-medical problems preventing discharge as well as being clever doctors (41). The same journal published replies from six geriatricians in following weeks (42, 43, 44, 45, 46 47). Their comments included the need to improve geriatric nursing expertise on acute wards, the satisfaction to be gained by using medical and other skills to help elderly patients, the bringing in to geriatrics of doctors from other specialties, and combined general/geriatric physician posts, the need to meet the growing demands of the elderly population, and the fact that geriatrics is general medicine whether it is at its best or worst.

To sum up: there are major differences between the experience and attitudes of geriatricians and non-geriatricians. We need to provide the best possible care for old people whichever hospital department they are in. We need to abolish the misconceptions and faulty thinking behind a referral note saying: 'This ninety-five year old senile woman was admitted two months ago with a stroke. She is not incontinent but cannot go home again. Could you please see her about transfer to one of your wards?'

2.8. *Information services*

These are the equivalent in resource organization terms of laboratories, X-ray, and ECG departments in individual patient care.

Many clinicians in and out of hospital have been reluctant to accept the need for a cost-benefit approach in the NHS. They sometimes feel it might lead to adverse criticism of their abilities, and deprive patients of the benefits of a free-choice situation. Some form of positive management is needed if only to establish that the care of individual patients is the best that can be achieved in the circumstances. This implies an analysis of the availability, cost, and effectiveness of various forms of management. For example, where different patient-support systems (beds) are available, how expensive are they, are they comfortable to lie in and will they prevent or reduce the incidence of pressure-sores? If the best equipment, buildings, staff, and the like, cannot be provided because they are too expensive or unobtainable, then cost-effective analysis should help select the next best management alternative.

In simple terms good management is saying what you want, and what you need to get what you want done without waste (48). There is a danger that the inadequate amount of money allocated to the NHS will lead to a more efficient use of resources, or even to the use of cheaper and fairly efficient alternatives, but at the cost of neglecting the effectiveness of the methods used. A cheap and rapid commercial laundry service may supplant a hospital laundry: 'efficiency'. This could be at the cost of more rapid deterioration of garments and a loss of flame-proofing, and of more pressure sores because of increased skin damage from toughened fabric, retention of detergent in the fabric, and an altered pH: 'ineffectiveness'.

Medical audit is not only a necessary response to insufficient money and rising costs but should also be seen as a way of ensuring that we are doing the best for our patients and are regularly reviewing our performance and adapting to changes in patient need and new methods of management. We cannot do this as individuals without help from colleagues.

This is an issue vital to all health and welfare services, and there have recently been several views of the methods and results of auditing medical care (49, 50). Some examples of beneficial managerial 'interference' in respect of care of the elderly have also been described (51, 52). They include an influenza epidemic in the staff of an acute teaching hospital forcing a rapid realization that there was a gross deficiency of geriatric beds. A fortuitous benefit was the finding that 75 per cent of laundry facilities were still needed even when no routine work was being carried out; this evidence was produced when an industrial dispute of ancillary workers led to a threat to reduce the laundry output to 25 per cent of normal, which was what the unions had believed to be the minimum to maintain essential services. Another example was a decision to set up a terminal care centre. Analysis of the needs, and ways of meeting them, became necessary after a charitable institution closed. It was decided that a purpose-built unit was the best replacement.

These are examples of effective responses to crises, but it is often much more difficult to get more routine matters examined by executive and planning committees. One excuse has been that information services are only at an embryo stage, and some of the few existing operational research units are research rather than service orientated. There are, however, many existing facilities which could provide Cogwheel divisions, family practitioner committees, community physicians, health care planning and district management teams with considerable information. These range from bed-usage figures on the geriatrician's office wall, and Hospital Activity Analyses, to the risk register developed by some GPs and the District Profiles already compiled by social service departments and health care planning teams for the elderly.

3. THE PROBLEM LIST

This is obtained by combining the data base of past history (1.1–1.8) with the examination of the present state of the 'patient' (2.1–2.7). Some positive future problems, as yet unconsidered, can also be added to the list. Problem listing is intended to clarify and facilitate management of each problem separately, but many problems in the elderly overlap and they are listed in groups. Problem solving (or inactivating) may require the acquisition of additional information, the provision of general or specific treatment, and education of the 'patient'.

3.1. *The 'problems' list*

I. GENERAL DEFECTS OF HEALTH AND SOCIAL SERVICES

(*a*) Low level of national and local spending.
(*b*) Disproportionate allocation of money and resources: for example, staffing, buildings, equipment, away from areas of need.
(*c*) Disproportionate geographical allocation of money and resources.
(*d*) Disproportionate allocation of money and resources between hospital, GP, community services.
(*e*) Defective standards of care.

II. CHANGING POPULATIONS; MORE OLD PEOPLE

(*f*) More physical problems in old age.
(*g*) More mental problems in old age.
(*h*) More social problems in old age.
(*i*) More mixed problems in old age.

III. EDUCATION. ATTITUDES. RESEARCH

(*j*) Defective education of medical students.
(*k*) Defective education of doctors.
(*l*) Defective education of other careers.
(*m*) Defective education of 'consumers' of all ages.
(*n*) Wrong and obstructive attitudes.

IV. GERIATRIC AND OTHER SERVICES FOR THE ELDERLY

(*o*) Geriatrics 'against' general medicine.
(*p*) Hospital/GP/community services.
(*q*) Staff deficiencies in geriatrics.

V. MONEY (*a–e*, see above)

(*r*) Inadequate pensions.

VI. INFORMATION SERVICES

(*s*) Defective nationally/internationally.
(*t*) Defective locally.
(*u*) Defective monitoring.
(*v*) Research in geriatrics.

VII. 'NEW' PROBLEM AREAS

(*w*) Insufficient doctors.
(*x*) Unforeseen medical developments.
(*y*) Unforeseen problems.
(*z*) Prevention of ill-health.

4. THE FUTURE

The problem list (section 3) is a daunting one, especially as it is incomplete. Many of the twenty-six problems listed are multiple and some are insoluble. Some have been discussed in some detail already, and possible solutions have been suggested. The problems of providing a comprehensive system for the care of old people are only part of the wider difficulties of a health service which is trying to do too much with too little, and doing it unfairly.

4.1. *General defects of health and social services* (Problems *a–e*)

Solution to problems: spend more money on these services, spend it more equitably and raise the pension considerably. If we want an unrestricted service we shall have to pay for it, and also accept a possible diversion of manpower and materials from other fields. If we cannot achieve an unrestricted service the general public will not be able to expect even the present help they get with looking after disabled elderly people.

The consumer demanding a better service and even being prepared to pay for it, should realize how the costs of personal services are soaring. 'Hotel' rather than medical items account for the astronomical cost of keeping patients in hospital. The average weekly cost per in-patient in an acute hospital in 1972–3 ranged from £81 at its cheapest to almost £130 at its most expensive (53). Many in-patients are elderly, and are in effect being paid for mainly by revenue raised from younger people.

In-patient costs also raise the issue of whether a choice of hospital versus non-hospital care can be decided entirely by patient need. Would it be cheaper to keep an old person out of hospital by organizing supportive services, even though life might be less happy or safe? Conversely, the high cost and difficulty of getting relatives and staff to support frail old people out of hospital (home help, meals-on-wheels service daily, expensive equipment and laundry) might make hospital the better alternative. The elderly persons involved also has some right to choose whether they should remain in a protected environment, and whether their own home is a sad or happy alternative to continued care in hospital or at home.

The difficulty of getting staff might prove a stumbling block even if more money could be injected into geriatrics. This objection is not entirely valid if only because material improvement in buildings and equipment would attract staff. On the debit side one certainly can say that the extra financial 'lead' for geriatric, and psychiatric, nurses has not corrected chronic staff shortages. The lead is a small one, and in any case the shortages may be more a consequence of poor buildings, wrong attitudes, and defective education (4.3).

Low income is also quoted as a cause of inadequate recruitment of doctors into geriatrics. There is little scope for private practice in geriatrics as most old people cannot pay for the long-term multidisciplinary team approach often needed. Few well-off old people, or their relatives, could afford it either. Most private insurance schemes exclude this sort of care, or severely limit the time for which they will pay benefits.

Nearly all geriatric physicians work wholetime in the NHS, but are able to add to their income and superannuation rights by domiciliary visiting. An annual ceiling of 300 paid visits is being established, but to achieve the maximum quota would occupy a considerable amount of a geriatrician's time. These visits can be invaluable in assessing patients in their own home, and often help to decide on the right course of action: admit to hospital, arrange out-patient or day-hospital attendance, or advise the GP on management. One wonders whether critical 'auditing' would show that a fair number are unnecessary, or could have been dealt with in some other way by GP–hospital–social service liaison. A feature of a geriatrician's work is travelling: to the various hospitals where his beds are located, to day-hospitals and clinics, and to giving specialist advice in hospital, homes, and at home. Mileage allowances are usually paid for much of this travelling and are increased at intervals, but even before petrol, servicing, and repair costs soared in 1973–4, many geriatricians were considerably out of pocket if they fulfilled their service commitments! Travelling expenses are also of concern to other hospital staff and GPs, but there is no way a geriatrician can avoid this monetary loss. A recent draft advertisement for a consultant geriatric post stipulated that whoever was appointed *must* provide his own transport.

Another bone of contention is the distribution of merit awards. Even if many geriatricians are not special enough to merit an award a total of eighteen new awards (54) in England and Wales (twelve in category C) is disproportionately low in relation to the number of hardworking and above-average doctors in the geriatric field. In many ways these awards are invidious, and are not being used for the purpose for which they were created, but while the system exists they should be distributed more fairly.

4.2. *Changing populations: more old people* (Problems *f–i*)

Statistical predictions of our future aged population are thought to be reasonably reliable. There may be half a million more retired people (women over 60, men over 65) in the year 2000 (2), many will be aged 75 plus, and there may be 200,000 more over-85s (1). They may have different attitudes to old age, and have been able to effect a better response to their needs. During the next thirty years, however, we are almost certainly going to be faced with an expanded geriatric 'problem'. Any breakthrough (4.7) in disease prevention (control of cancer, arteriosclerosis, or arthritis) or modification of 'ageing' will almost certainly take several generations to show its effect.

(*f*) Four common representative problems of old age, that will probably become more common, will now be discussed. They have emotional and social implications, are often multifactorial in their aetiology, and may coexist with or contribute to several other problems in the same patient.

(i) Incontinence. This is usually urinary. Faecal incontinence can cause even more distress. Incontinence should not be dismissed as due to senility, and a full history and careful examination are indicated in every case. An effective, reliable, accurate, and acceptable method of urine collection is needed to obtain specimens for bacteriological examination in appropriate cases. Midstream and catheter specimens, and supra-pubic aspirates often do not meet these requirements. More sophisticated investigations, such as cystometrography, may be indicated.

Incontinence often coexists with, and may be caused or

aggravated by, other conditions, for example, locomotor disability, constipation, ingestion of diuretics, mental impairment. It may also be caused by the logistics of just existing: if it takes an in-patient an average of two minutes to get to a lavatory and pass urine, and there are two lavatories in a ward for twenty-five patients, some patients will almost certainly be incontinent after a meal.

Some of the deficiencies and simple remedies available have been investigated by the Disabled Living Foundation (55). Incontinent old people can often be helped, but for those who remain incontinent an inexpensive, reliable and acceptable appliance is needed. An effective invention would benefit a tremendous number of people and would be the equivalent of a breakthrough such as the opening clip on shoe polish tins or cat's-eyes in the roads. An indwelling catheter may not work, often introduces infection, and is a remarkably immobilizing and humiliating imposition for a person of any age.

(ii) Strokes. Almost three-quarters of the 130,000 stroke victims living in private households have severe, or very severe, disability (57), and 18,000 hospital beds a day are occupied by elderly patients with cerebral vascular diseases, the majority having suffered strokes (21). This occupancy represented one-fifth of the geriatric beds and of the medical beds occupied by over-65s, and one-tenth of all medical beds, excluding maternity and psychiatry. It has been suggested that GPs have 5–10 new stroke patients yearly, in addition to 5–10 already in their practice.

The needs of these old people, from the time they develop their stroke until they are rehabilitated or die, are poorly served. They do not receive the medical or social recognition accorded to other handicapped groups. Where is the Stroke Society to rival the Multiple Sclerosis Society?

It has been suggested (57) that more epidemiological studies of strokes are needed, that better standard criteria of stroke assessment are required, that services for stroke disability need improving in every respect, that studies of different methods of treatment are required, and that some specialized stroke units should be established. These could explore all the areas suggested, and would almost certainly improve the lot of stroke patients admitted to them.

(iii) Pressure sores. These are all too common in elderly patients, cause great pain and suffering, and are expensive in bed-occupancy, nursing, and money. It has been suggested that hospital treatment of pressure sores costs £60,000,000 annually in the UK (58). There is insufficient collaboration between nurses and doctors in the management of pressure areas. Unproven myth often lies behind a nursing record of 'pressure areas treated'. Medical default often forces nurses to treat pressure areas and established sores with highly personal, and often bizarre, combinations of washing, friction, and topical applications. Lotio rubra, Friar's balsam, honey, insulin, and draughts of oxygen, have all been mentioned to me and the way their selection varies from nurse to nurse and week to week is an indictment of our lack of a positive and proven approach.

Simple principles apply to the management of fragile skin and pressure sores:

(*a*) Identify the at-risk patient (old, immobile, incontinent, very fat or very thin, confused, ill, and malnourished).

(*b*) Spread the pressure load (turning by nurses—even when 'asleep'—and patient-support systems).

(*c*) Keep the skin clean, but with a minimum of irritating medicaments or dressings (washing, catheterizing, topical applications).

(*d*) Improve the general health of the patient (correct anaemia, avoid excessive sedation, give appropriate physiotherapy).

Those dealing with the elderly wherever they are should review their methods of preventing pressure sores as well as their management of established sores. A general medical-nursing approach should be established. A great deal more research is needed into nursing techniques (59), the comparative benefits of support systems (60), the benefits and demerits of topical applications and general measures including the place of vitamin C and zinc supplements.

Pressure sores can even be annoying after death. If they are entered on a death certificate an inquest almost inevitably follows. They clearly can be a cause of death, but most doctors probably try and certify some other cause which had acted terminally, rather than inconvenience relatives and staff.

(*g*) Dementia/confusion. Almost half the psychiatric hospital beds are occupied by the over-65s, and the number of elderly people admitted to psychiatric hospitals is rising. Despite the burden of caring for mentally impaired old people, relatives, friends, and community services still cope with most elderly dements. The predicted increase in the elderly population with its extra group of dements carries the threat that 'we can certainly not take it for granted that the fine balance between home and institutional care on which services now depend will endure' (61).

Depression and confusion are common concomitants of dementia, and some insight can be retained even in moderately severe dementia. The remorselessness with which dementia leads to mental incapacity and loss of dignity probably causes as much or more physical and mental stress for the beholder as for the victim. The indignities of dementia and confusion are probably a major factor in people's attitudes to old age. Much can be done to help elderly dements, and exclude and minimize other mental problems. Once again, a positive approach is needed to identify the need, place it in perspective in the over-all picture of health resource needs, and provide the most appropriate methods of coping with the need.

Prevention of dementia and the possibility of preventing or reversing failing intellect in established dementia has become a 'growth-market' for pharmaceutical companies. Many medicaments are available to try and increase cerebral blood flow or to enhance the performance of surviving brain cells, but it is difficult to find any proven evidence of benefit from these drugs. It may be that investigations not yet available will show marginal deficiencies of vitamins, electrolytes, or trace elements in 'dementia' which can then be called confusion, and that appropriate supplements would be beneficial. Investigations might also prove that the metabolic efficiency of normal or 'ageing' brain cells could be improved with an arrest or reversal of mental impairment. Any of these methods should theoretically be able to improve intellectual ability in non-demented people.

The basic problem of dementia still remains. Brain cells have died, the person is not so good mentally as he was, and the process cannot be reversed. Prevention of brain cell death might come by control of arteriosclerosis, discovery of the cause of the idiopathic 'chronic brain syndrome' or from general anti-ageing treatments (4.6, 4.7).

4.3. *Education. Attitudes. Research* (Problems *j–n*)

Geriatrics is not a classification of people by age or disease but a whole skilled philosophy, to paraphrase Lord Amulree. In hospital practice it is not a service to take elderly patients away somewhere else once other doctors have had a go at them, and failed to look after them. Changes are needed in education about old age not just to improve the attitudes and skills of health service personnel, but also for the general public. Some of the senior boys at my eldest son's school do a great amount of voluntary work with the elderly, but for most of them it is as an alternative to games. Well under half of the boys see their grandparents regularly, and many think that people over 30 are old.

(*j*) Adequate education about old age should be an essential part of basic medical education. The General Medical Council has stated that a student should be given 'a comprehensive understanding of man in health and in sickness and an intimate acquaintance with his physical and social environment' (62). The GMC has also emphasized the 'increasing importance of the problems of disability and disease in an ageing population'. The main purpose of education is to give the student the skills to do his work properly, but exposure to good geriatric practice should also increase recruitment into geriatrics. It would be wrong of the DHSS or geriatricians to suggest to the GMC education committee that it should put a greater obligation on medical schools to emphasize the importance of geriatrics in an effort to fill vacant geriatric posts. It would be eminently right to suggest it to correct glaring educational deficiencies.

Most medical schools have accepted that three other important aspects of medicine should be given due acknowledgement. Psychiatry, child health, and community medicine are being given substantial recognition in most undergraduate curricula and in-course and examination assessment. It is to be hoped that similar progress will occur in the teaching of geriatric medicine.

(*k–n*) There is also a need for continuing education in all fields of medicine. An encouraging feature of British practice has been the growth of the postgraduate movement. The Royal Colleges are also increasingly setting standards for postgraduate training (63). It is clear that geriatric experience would be an acceptable part of general professional training. Higher training for geriatric specialists would benefit from secondments into other specialties such as psychiatry and general practice (64). Rotation at pre-registration and senior house officer and registrar level would also benefit trainees whether or not they become geriatricians.

Some geriatric departments might be helped by the DHSS to become centres to investigate educational experiments such as schemes rotating geriatric registrars into general practice. These 'centres of excellence' should not deprive other geriatric departments of normal support. They could also prove that displays of equipment, and medical, nursing, and other training courses and research could be successfully organized in every district. They might also investigate what doctors really need in the way of on-going education to improve their clinical performance, and how those doctors who do not come forward at present could be persuaded to accept further education.

It might be that we need to accredit hospitals, rather than individual posts, for their educational worth. The American Joint Commission for Hospital Accreditation is responsible for approving hospitals for postgraduate education. This led to the Commission examining and setting standards for long-stay institutions. We do have standards of staffing and material provision for geriatric wards but these are minimal and have little impact on the image of geriatrics or its educational role. Our Hospital Advisory Service has done a great job in examining individual geriatric departments. In the future it, or its regional or area successors, should make an effort to help the DHSS lay down general standards for geriatric departments.

4.4. *Geriatrics and other services* (Problems *o–p*)

(*o*) The number and multiple problems of old people in any DGH, its branch community hospitals, and its district might best be served by deciding that some consultant physician posts falling vacant should be redesignated for geriatric medicine. The new geriatrician would retain some, or all, of the beds and facilities (in the DGH) of his predecessor. He would complement the work of any geriatrician(s) in post in that area by helping with more old people in the hospital and the local community. This suggestion would probably work best if the post altered had been fairly general in its medical scope as the hospital would then retain its quota of 'specialists'.

More geriatricians are also needed to continue the impetus of established geriatric care, to maintain specialized liaison between hospital and other parts of the health and social services, to teach and to do research. Local experiments, such as orthopaedic–geriatric liaison or a five-day ward, could be expanded and other innovations tested. Geriatrics should not stand still: if it can get more recruits there is a great need for specialists to see more old people in non-geriatric wards, mental hospitals, and out of hospital. A major, but rewarding exercise, would be to help GPs to screen elderly at-risk populations such as those asking for welfare home admission, or already in homes. We might even challenge the role of homes as hotels for the elderly. It is probable that we shall see a swing away from hospitals in the future, and the primary care role of the GP will become even more important. General practitioners may be even more useful than they are now in helping to cope with elderly people in hospital by continuing to help to look after their own patients after admission, or by staffing the longer-stay wards.

The brunt of geriatric work falls on nurses, social workers, other professions allied to medicine, friends and relatives as much as on GPs and geriatricians. It has been suggested (65) that geriatricians should give up some clinical commitments, increase their contacts with these other people and give more time to teaching and administration. Most geriatricians like seeing their patients and feel that they should be clinically available to be 'responsible' for them. An additional danger of this approach is that it produces the worst sort of 'Professor'—teaching, researching, and administering in a vacuum.

(*p*) How much can other personnel help the GP to deal with the elderly? A multidisciplinary team attached to a group practice working in a health centre is an obvious and proven way of delivering comprehensive services in densely populated districts. There is no reason why some form of GP partnership and team approach should not also be effective in rural districts. Where GPs are in a group, or even loosely linked, there is a lot to be said for one having special training and responsibility for the elderly in the area, and possibly a hospital attachment. There could be dangers in all GPs becoming narrow specialists but a geriatric GP would be an invaluable asset.

A nurse-practitioner might be a useful innovation in under-doctored and sparsely populated areas. A Canadian study (66) has suggested that, with additional training, a nurse can become a 'co-practitioner'. These nurses' roles went far beyond those of a community nurse or health visitor. This type of person might also help in the preventive approach by organizing a general practice risk register. With efficient, problem-oriented, note-keeping a register could produce two types of benefits for the elderly. Those most at risk (very old, single, poor, disabled, and affected by multiple disorders) could be seen regularly and independence maintained as long as possible. Those at particular risk (the same group plus people with certain specific disorders) could be seen as soon as possible at times of crisis. Examples of a crisis might be bereavement, or a cold spell and fuel strike, when people generally at-risk but who had also recovered from hypothermia previously, or were taking chlorpromazine, would be at extra risk. The actions necessary to apply the benefits of registering the aged would often need considerable social work help and it has been suggested that risk registers might best be kept by social service departments.

One of the unsolved problems in registering old people is that of confidentiality. When medical and social details are available or given to non-medical and even volunteer staff, it is all to easy to omit getting the patient's permission. Another problem is the difficulty of locating and helping some of those most in need, such as people who have not seen a doctor for a long time or are not even on a doctor's list.

The GP, or social service team could also use the register to select old people for specialist attention. This screening would find groups of people with potentially easily remediable disorders of hearing, sight, teeth, feet, and mental function.

A home care organizer might be a useful new 'grade' to help to marry up all the personal services available for the elderly. She could help to match need to provision and co-ordinate meals-on-wheels, home helps, laundry services, community nursing, provision of specialized equipment, and the use of voluntary help.

Supporting services are often needed for old people in sheltered housing. This is usually purpose-built and often has a warden who helps to supervise the services provided and is available in times of crisis. This sort of accommodation may be one of the main ways of meeting future demand. Although not needing many staff (otherwise it would become an expensive 'home') they would often need more immediate support than the one or two wardens for forty of fifty flats, which is normal in England. Sheltered housing could also be included in new council and private housing developments, with only half-a-dozen special flats on each estate. Even more speculative is a suggestion that specially designed accommodation might be developed for people to move to in middle age, which would enable the majority to remain there for the rest of their lives.

Welfare homes should provide for old people whose needs fall between sheltered accommodation and hospital. They have become progressively smaller and more pleasant, often with individual rooms and space for personal belongings. They also tend to admit frailer and older people than in the past, and to keep residents there as long as possible even if they deteriorate. Unfortunately they too often present an image like a modern airport lounge with rather apathetic travellers sitting about waiting for the next meal or departure. The present provision and future plans for old people's homes really do need urgent review to see if we can prove that we are doing the right thing and doing it properly. A few places have successfully developed homes that cater for residents who are very frail from the time of admission, and also serve as a day-centre and luncheon club for fitter old people living nearby.

Careful experiments challenging accepted methods are to be welcomed. We spent more than £50 million on residential care in 1970–1. There is little evidence that we have satisfactorily explored alternatives to homes or alternative types or ways of using homes. If old people are good enough to be accepted into the 'hotel' of an old people's home, why are they going there at all? Permanent care in a home or hospital may be a better 'Last Refuge' than it was in 1960 (67), but institutions still find it difficult to be homes. Residential homes for the elderly are legally intended to be for people in need of care and protection. Only a few residents ever leave and re-establish an independent existence. A few are only in the home for a 'holiday break' to help relatives, but even some of these join the permanent residents.

Progressive authorities do try to provide some stimulus to rehabilitation with occupational therapy, physiotherapy, and other interests. All too often this is 'diversionary' and passes the time of day, and does not provide an atmosphere of 'improvement' rehabilitation. There are almost 2,000 private homes (not nursing homes) in the country with an estimated 24,000 residents. These homes may provide even less of a therapeutic and rehabilitative atmosphere.

Some geriatricians have had formal links with local authorities, and many have established friendly informal links. There is clearly a great need to increase these links to provide specialized advice and even some clinical expertise in the 'community'. A few geriatricians have already been able to liaise effectively with the social workers and GPs involved with the residents of old people's homes, and with the staff of the homes. If this could be widely introduced (depending on the availability of geriatricians, and sympathetic attitudes all round) it might lead to a more thorough medical screening of applicants for admission and a more organized approach to problems in the homes such as confusion, incontinence, and polypharmacy. Another priority is the need to review our provisions for the elderly mentally infirm: and try to decide whether residential homes should admit them. If they should, would it be best to mix them with, or separate them from, mentally normal people however physically disabled they are?

These are all matters for district health care planning teams to examine, although many of them would merit careful consideration at area, regional, and national level.

(*q*) The problems of staff deficiencies mentioned in 1.4 (education), 1.6 (psycho-geriatrics), 1.7 (attitudes), 2.2 (hospital services) 2.5 (staffing), 2.6 (money), and 2.7 (geriatrics versus general medicine) and their solutions are usually self-evident. Pay more money, improve working conditions, educate health service personnel and consumer, use existing facilities as well as possible and look for new methods of caring. If this could be achieved then medical students and doctors might realize that 'a career in geriatrics is an attractive proposition, with its range of problems, prospects of consultant appointment at an early age for doctors of both sexes, and a virtual guarantee that they will never be out of a job, and may be enhancing the outlook for their own old age' (3).

4.5. *Money* (Problems *a–e*, *r*)

(*a–e*) The problems of inadequate spending on staff and resources have already been discussed (2.6, 4.1).

(*r*) The need for a higher pension and regular substantial increases has been stated but another important point must be made. It is necessary to distinguish between providing a substantial pension with little or no supplementation and a medium pension with considerable supplements for those who 'need' them. The theoretical average of both systems might be the same but the second might lead to a much lower take-up rate in practice. The Treasury must be thankful that all those eligible for supplementary benefits do not claim them (7). Non-claiming might be mainly because of not knowing about eligibility, but also because of pride or lethargy. Of course a much higher pension might improve social well-being without much gain in health in old age. This is unlikely, but an old person might choose to spend a higher pension on 'luxuries' rather than good food, accommodation, heating, and clothing.

This is not an advocacy of unbridled ever-increasing spending on health and social services. A big spender should still put the money to its maximum use and a modern and evolving administrative machinery is needed to spend the money wisely. A relatively costly and centrally funded NHS is needed to cater for the needs of the elderly, as well as effective local reorganization. A substantial pension rise would not give old people the spending power to pay for health care. The current consumption of health services by the elderly is probably a major argument against a large-scale return to 'private' medicine.

4.6. *Information services* (Problems *s–v*)

(*s–t*) We need to improve fact-finding and cost-effectiveness analysis. The sort of question one needs to ask is:

(i) Is it cheaper: more acceptable, and healthier for disabled old people to be in hospital, home, sheltered accommodation, or supported at home?

(ii) Are our methods of managing incontinence, confusion, stroke, and pressure sores the best?

The word 'best' or phrase 'optimal care' must be used cautiously. The best may not be necessary for everybody, might be hopelessly wasteful, and not even acceptable to proud independent old people. We would not benefit every 80-year-old with congestive cardiac failure by investigating with chest X-ray, electrocardiogram, urea, electrolytes, and serum digoxin assay, treating with digoxin, diuretic, potassium supplement, and salt restriction, and keeping them in hospital to make sure they receive their medicines.

We need to improve the dissemination of knowledge already gained. The findings of a study showing that simple measures can reduce urinary incontinence in homes and hospitals might very well have been done, perhaps by a geriatrician in the north of Scotland. The results might have been published in a specialist journal, and even rated a paragraph in a newspaper. The conclusions might not reach the rest of the country, or someone else might do the same research, unless national and local information systems are geared to feeding such findings into their own plans and provisions. Area and district medical and administrative staff have an important role to play in this respect.

(*u*) These staff will also have to monitor performance as well as help spread knowledge. Meals-on-wheels supplied to those in need are meant to provide calories and vitamins for those who are unable to obtain sufficient satisfactory meals for themselves; social contact is a subsidiary function. It was perhaps lucky that one local authority was only able to supply meals on two days of the week as in some aspects the meals supplied were less nutritious than the food eaten on the non-meals-on-wheels days (68).

(*s*) An 'International Federation on Ageing' has recently been formed which will provide a global forum for discussing problems of ageing and retirement planning. It will be in the unique position of comparing the different achievements of different countries in providing services for the elderly. In 'Denmark it's the housing concept, in Sweden it's home delivered services, in Russia it's an extensive research programme' (69). The mention of retirement planning is interesting as there is considerable evidence that people can still learn, and enjoy, a wide range of new activities in middle and old age. In spite of present financial crises more leisure and earlier retirement can be expected in years to come. If we really can become more prosperous, perhaps from North Sea resources, we may be able to indulge in more extra-mural classes and opportunities for hobbies and entertainment in old age.

(*v*) Research is another aspect of information seeking. We have no Gerontological Research Institute, nor do we have a Post-graduate Centre of any kind in geriatrics. A great deal of research has been carried out by service geriatricians. Much of it is cross-sectional and being based on local experience may have limited wider application. The Glasgow 'school' of geriatrics has a reputation for careful and useful cross-sectional and longitudinal research but even they have not really ventured to initiate geriatric research starting in youth or middle age. Breakdown may tend to start after 70 but diseases causing breakdown (vascular disease, neoplasia, arthritis) begin at a much younger age. More longitudinal research would also be able to assess the complex effects of the interplay of social factors, such as social class, marital status, and education, with medical factors, such as smoking, obesity, and diabetes mellitus. North American and Scandinavian studies may be revealing when the population cohorts under review become old, but they may have been recording unrewarding parameters and omitting important uses. Gerontological ageing research should not only suggest ways of prolonging healthy life, but might reveal ways in which established degenerative, neoplastic, and disabling disorders might be minimized in old age.

The worldwide use of the contraceptive pill has led to a reawakening of interest into the possible reduction of cardio-vascular and bone disease in post-menopausal women. Side-effects from the pill are at present balanced against the risks of pregnancy, and the pill comes off better. Can we compare the risks of thrombo-embolism and fluid retention, as seen in elderly men treated with oestrogens for prostatic cancer, against a possible reduction in the incidence of arterial disease of brain, heart, and legs, and of osteoporosis?

A relative lack of exercise over many years is thought to be one of the important factors in the causation of osteoporosis. Bones deprived of repeated periosteal 'stimulation' by muscle action rapidly rarefy. If more people took more sensible exercise from youth onwards we might see a remarkable reduction in the incidence of osteoporosis and of heart disease, always remembering that this could be at the expense of a reciprocal rise in the incidence of osteo-arthritis.

Lack of calcium and vitamin D may be involved in the causation of osteoporosis as well as osteomalacia. Thus we might radically reduce the incidence of bone disease in old age if we could establish the correct prophylactic 'doses' of oestrogens or androgens, of exercise, and of calcium and vitamin D, and when to start them. This sort of question has already been answered in some aspects of prophylaxis.

Another tantalizing mixture of knowledge and speculation concerns smoking. Two-fifths of heavy smokers, but only one-fifth of non-smokers, die before they are 65. If smokers can be persuaded to stop they often attain the same level of death-risk as non-smokers within ten years of stopping, if they live that long. If smoking could be reduced there would still be many sufferers from tobacco-linked diseases for some years to come. A cut in revenue from tobacco would considerably reduce national tax income now. This is not a 'justification' for spending so little on putting the case against smoking. Many very old people do not smoke, or have never smoked; so the effect of changing smoking habits might produce a whole new geriatric population. Similar tantalizing speculation surrounds the possibility of reducing ill-health from cardiovascular disease, by a combination of 'sensible' diet and exercise. This approach might also slow down the 'ageing' process.

What is really needed is a combined geriatric–gerontological approach considering long-term health-preserving measures and more immediate practical measures to prevent breakdown in old age (70). It is sad to read that the majority of very old people living alone in an Inner London borough were elderly ladies who were very poor, lived in bad accommodation, were seriously disabled, and physically could only manage to get through every day with great difficulty (71). Our research must be aimed at preventing this type of medical and social breakdown. Our tolerant (permissive) society may look to euthanasia to deal with some of these problems. A remarkable book by a medical priest (72) manages to encompass religious, agnostic, atheistic, antagonistic, and protagonistic views of euthanasia. The facts about dying are inescapable. What is uncertain is how we die and what happens afterwards if anything. We cannot necessarily control the latter but an expert and positive approach certainly can make the former better than it often is at present. Distress in the eye of the (non-aged) beholder is not necessarily a reason for permitting euthanasia, especially if the distress is amenable to treatment.

4.7. *New 'problem areas'* (Problems *w–z*)

(*w*) The possibility of a reduced number of foreign doctors has been discussed (2.5). Entry into the EEC may oblige us to increase the number of hours of medical training, with a reduction in the number of students trained. A reduction in the number of doctors might be coped with by increased efficiency and effectiveness, including redistribution of medical manpower into previously under-doctored specialites, and the use of non-medical personnel. An over-all increase in the number of doctors could come by expanding our existing medical schools and/or creating new ones: an open medical university?

(*x*) Unforeseen medical developments might alter the geriatric need. Current research on ageing suggests that the pathological biological clock can only be altered slowly. Increased life-expectation and better health in old age could come from accepting knowledge already gained (see 4.6), but would tend to benefit generations not yet old. It is possible there will be unexpected breakthroughs akin to the reduction or abolition in deaths due to infectious diseases that occurred in the late Victorian era. Thousands of deaths in children and young adults were caused by measles, whooping-cough, diphtheria, gastro-enteritis, typhus, and smallpox.

Changes in other countries may precipitate changes in Western lives and in the numbers of old people, possibly by retarding improvements in health and life expectation. Examples are the increasing world populations: the need for more food, and economic pressures from individual groups such as the energy and raw material producers.

(*y*) Some 'hidden' problems may be clearly identifiable and their solution fairly obvious. Screening for ill-health should be aimed at disorders that can be easily found by simple methods without much interference with the subject. When found they should be able to be easily and cheaply remedied. Obvious examples in old age are disorders affecting:

(i) Eyes. The detection and treatment of cataract and simple chronic glaucoma, the assessment of visual deterioration, and the efficacy of refractive correction.

(ii) Ears. The updating of hearing aids to make them more efficient medically and socially acceptable, and the investigation of preventable causes of hearing loss (pop music?).

(iii) Teeth. The provision of effective dentures and effective dental services to prevent dental decay and unnecessary extraction. The majority of old people living now had all their teeth extracted in youth or middle age.

(iv) Locomotor disability. Ranging from the need for better chiropody services to techniques for restoring mobility to stroke victims. This might be by more corrective surgery or powered equipment or even power assistance connected into disabled limbs.

(*7*) The prevention of ill-health is paramount in geriatrics. To adapt one of Marjory Warren's sayings, life should not only be longer but easier. This will need a change in beliefs, attitudes, and the amount of money we are prepared to spend.

REFERENCES

1. Royal College of Physicians of London (1972). *Report of the College Committee on Geriatric Medicine.*
2. Office of Population Censuses and Surveys (1973). *Population Projections 3 1972–2012* (London: HMSO).
3. Green, M. F. (1973). *Br. J. Hosp. Med.* 12, 672.
4. Weed, L. L. (1969). *Medical Records, Medical Education, and Patient Care* (Cleveland, Ohio: Press of Case Western Reserve University).
5. Williamson, J., *et al.* (1964). *Lancet*, ii, 1117.
6. Department of Health and Social Security and Ministry of Housing and Local Government (1970). Joint Circular, *DHSS Circular 12/70* (London: HMSO).
7. Fox, R. H., *et al.* (1973). *Br. med. J.* 1, 200.
8. Datta, S. B., and Andrews, C. T. (1973). *Gerontologia Clinica*, 15, 181.
9. Department of Health and Social Security (1972). *Services for the Elderly with Mental Illness* (London: HMSO).

10. ANDREWS, J., *et al.* (1972). *Gerontologia Clinica*, 14, 100.
11. BAKER, A. A. (1974). *Lancet*, ii, 795.
12. BAKER, A. A. (1973). *Modern Geriatrics*, 9, 471.
13. GALE, J., and LIVESLEY, B. (1974). *Age and Aging*, 3, 49.
14. TOWNSEND, P. (1974). *Lancet*, ii, 1181.
15. HALL, M. R. P. (1974). *Medicine*, 25, 1465.
16. FERGUSON ANDERSON, SIR W. (1974). Leader, *Modern Geriatrics*, 4,294.
17. *Hospital Advisory Service Annual Report of 1972* (1973). (London: HMSO).
18. KUSHLICK, A. (1972). *The Elderly Mind* (British Hospital Journal/ Hospital International UK).
19. EXTON-SMITH, A. N., and MILLARD, P. H. (1973). Paper presented at DHSS/BGS Conference on the Care of the Elderly.
20. SUTHERLAND, A. (1972). *A Study of Long Stay Admissions to the Acute Medical Wards of the Aberdeen Hospitals* (Edinburgh: Scottish Home and Health Department).
21. HUNT, L. V. (1973). *Br. med. J.* 4, 83.
22. MCKEOWN, P. (1960). *Report of the 10th National Conference on Care of the Elderly* (London: National Old Peoples' Welfare Council).
23. THOMPSON, M. K. (1974). *Modern Geriatrics*, 7, 262.
24. SIDEL, V. W., *et al.* (1972). *Jl R. Coll. Gen. Practit.* 22, supplement 3.
25. AGE CONCERN (1972) *Age Concern Today*. issue 1, spring 1972 (see also subsequent issues).
26. MEACHER, M. (1972). *Taken For A Ride* (London: Longman).
27. DEPARTMENT OF HEALTH AND SOCIAL SECURITY (1973). Statistics and Research Division, *National Tables of Hospital Medical Staff* (London: HMSO).
28. BRITISH GERIATRIC SOCIETY (1971). *Memorandum of Unfilled Posts in Geriatrics.*
29. *On the State of the Public Health: Annual Report of the Chief Medical Officer of the DHSS* (1972). (London: HMSO).
30. COCHRANE, A. L. (1971). *Effectiveness and Efficiency*. Rock Carling Monograph (London: Nuffield Provincial Hospitals Trust).
31. NATIONAL CORPORATION FOR THE CARE OF OLD PEOPLE (1973). *Housing in Retirement* (London).
32. DROLLER, H. (1974). *Modern Geriatrics*, 6, 250.
33. LLOYD, C. M. (1970). *RCP Report of Pilot Survey into Mental Impairment in the Elderly* (London: Royal College of Physicians).
34. PRITCHARD, J. G. (1961). *Gerontologia Clinica*, 3, 220.
35. DEPARTMENT OF HEALTH AND SOCIAL SECURITY (1973). *National Symposium on the Care of the Dying* (London: HMSO).

36. Brocklehurst, J. C. (1970). *The Geriatric Day Hospital* (King Edward's Hospital Fund for London).
37. de Largy, K. (1957). *Lancet*, i, 418.
38. Isaacs, B., and Thompson, J. (1960). Ibid. i, 969.
39. Parnell, J. W., and Naylor, R. (1973). *Home for the Weekend—Back on Monday* (Queen's Institute of District Nursing).
40. Leading article (1974). *Lancet*, ii, 663.
41. Crockett, V. S. (1974). Ibid. ii, 805.
42. Coni, N. K. (1974). Ibid. ii, 924.
43. Millard, P. H. (1974). Ibid. ii, 925.
44. Staffurth, J. S. (1974). Ibid. ii, 985.
45. Charatan, F. B. (1974). Ibid. ii, 986.
46. Hyams, D. E. (1974). Ibid. ii, 1234.
47. Todd, J. W. (1973). Ibid. ii, 1106.
48. Maxwell, R. (1973). *Br. med. J.* 1, 160.
49. *British Medical Journal* (1974). Leading article, 1, 255.
50. *British Medical Journal* (1974). 'Contemporary themes', 1, 271.
51. Department of Health and Social Security (1974). *Joint Working Party on the Organization of Medical Work in Hospitals* (Cogwheel) (London: HMSO).
52. Joint Working Party on the Organization of Medical Work in Hospitals (1974). *Information for Action* (London: HMSO).
53. Department of Health and Social Security (1974). *Hospital Costing Returns for 1972–3* (London: HMSO).
54. British Medical Journal (Supplement) (1974). *Distribution of New Distinction Awards*, 3575, 75.
55. Disabled Living Foundation (1973). *Management of Incontinence in the Home: A summary of the results of a survey* (London).
56. Harris, A. I., Cox, E., and Smith, C. R. W. (1971). *Handicapped and Impaired in Great Britain*, Part I. Office of Population Censuses and Surveys (London: HMSO).
57. *Personal Communication (1974). Report of the Geriatrics Committee Working Group on Strokes* (London: Royal College of Physicians).
58. Fernie, G. R. (1973). PhD Thesis. University of Strathclyde.
59. Norton, D., McLaren, R., and Exton-Smith, A. N. (1962). *An Investigation of Geriatric Nursing Problems in Hospital* (London: National Corporation for the Care of Old People).
60. Redfern, S. J., Jeneid, P. A., Gillingham, M. E., and Lunn, H. F. (1973). *Lancet*, iii, 277.
61. Arie, T. (1973). In Canvin, R. W., and Pearson, N. G. (eds), *Needs of the Elderly* (University of Exeter).
62. General Medical Council (1967). *Recommendations as to Basic Medical Education.*

63. Royal College of Physicians, Royal College of General Practitioners (1973). *Report of the Joint Committee on General Professional Training* (London).

64. Royal College of Physicians (1972). *The Joint Committee on Higher Medical Training. First Report* (Edinburgh, Glasgow, Ireland, and London).

65. Wright, W. B. (1973). *Lancet*, iii, 252.

66. Spitzer, W. O., *et al.* (1974). *New Engl. J. Med.* 290, 251.

67. Townsend, P. (1960). *Last Refuge* (London: Routledge and Kegan Paul).

68. Davies, L., Hastrop, K., and Bender, A. E. (1973). *Modern Geriatrics*, 7, 390.

69. Viewpoint (1974). *Geriatrics*, 4, 46.

70. Brocklehurst, J. C. (1974). *Modern Geriatrics*, 7, 306.

71. Social Research Unit (1972). *Survey of Households and Individuals in Potential Need in the London Borough of Camden in 1969* (London: Bedford College).

72. Trowell, H. (1973). *The Unfinished Debate on Euthanasia* (SCM Press).

Psychiatry

COLIN GODBER

COLIN GODBER
BM, BCh, MRCP, MRCPsych
Psycho-geriatrician

Psychiatry

INTRODUCTION

I must preface this paper with one or two apologies. I have slanted my speculations on the future of psychiatry in the direction of my own views on the matter. This has resulted in my placing particular emphasis on issues about which decisions are being, or should be, made at the present time, and neglecting other important aspects. I have to admit to little practical experience in some of the fields on which I will discourse at some length, and must regret that my own area of interest has to be covered briefly because of its overlap with Dr Green's subject.

I have reduced to a minimum the punctuation of this paper by references, but will mention at this point a few of the important publications influencing the progress of psychiatry at present. Professor Denis Hill's Rock Carling Monograph, *Psychiatry in Medicine* (20) was an important landmark. There have been a number of DHSS Memoranda (1, 2, 3) on the future of the psychiatric services, as well as various asides on official policy by Dr Brothwood (6, 7, 13). A detailed appraisal of such planning (5), with further recommendations, was issued by a tripartite committee of the Royal College of Psychiatrists, the Society of Medical Officers of Health, and the British Medical Association, which emphasized some of the doubts which have been raised as to the norms emanating from the DHSS. The recent Nuffield Provincial Hospitals Trust publication *Policy for Action* (7) reported on the proceedings of a symposium in which this debate was carried further. This paper was largely completed before details of the laudable recommendations of the Trethowan Committee on the future role of the clinical psychologist (4) were available, and I have therefore given them less coverage than they merit. The Consultative Document was diplomatically cautious, and, in my view, still too subservient to the tradition that every referral to an NHS agency requires vetting by a doctor.

I shall be using the word 'psychiatry' rather loosely to denote the whole field of treatment of behaviour disorder, incorporating with this much of the sphere of influence of social workers and GPs, rather than the particular territory of the psychiatrist. Indeed my main theme is the need to organize a broad psychiatric service in which the specialist plays only a limited role in support of the generalist, as in no other way can I envisage society's potential case-load being handled. In the first section I shall describe some trends in psychiatry in relation to their influence on the future. I shall then go on to consider the main challenges to the services and how these may be met, and in particular how the 'psychiatric team' of the future might be deployed.

Trends in psychiatry

Psychiatry has moved in the last few decades from the provision of custodial care in remote institutions to an emphasis on community-based services and a general tone of therapeutic optimism. These advances have come about partly as a result of innovations in physical treatment notably the phenothiazines, electroconvulsive therapy (ECT), and the antidepressants, and partly through changes in attitudes within psychiatry which have led to the hospital milieu supporting rather than hindering recovery, and on the part of the public which have been mirrored by successive legislation designed to make it easier to get in and out of a hospital bed.

This trend is exemplified by the current migration of the acute psychiatric unit to the district general hospital (DGH), with which rather uneven progress has been made in the last twenty years. The hope is that these DGH units, working on much lower bed/population ratios than would have been dreamt possible in the 1950s, will be able to deal with the great majority of in-patient care in general psychiatry. They will have the advantage of proximity to the areas they serve and of day facilities to exploit this. One therefore envisages a much more flexible movement of patients between the three main areas of care (out-patient, day-care, in-patient), and, provided that other resources such as social workers, day centres, and hostels become available too, the goal of community care may become a reality. This latter proviso is, of course, an important one, as the last year or two has generally witnessed a sharp decline in the capacity of the social services to cope with their mental health responsibilities, though one looks forward to improvement as the teething problems of Seebohm and the social services departments settle down. I shall discuss later on how the manning of the community psychiatric services might be envisaged.

Patients will obviously continue to enter the 'long-stay' category but the work of Mann (21) suggests that many of these could be coped with adequately in hostels and small specialized hospital units backed by adequate day facilities. If the financial allocations to the health and social services ever catch up with the demand one might therefore anticipate the building of such units at the district level, though in the meantime one anticipates that in most areas the mental hospital will continue to serve that function. Just as the predictions of the 1962 Hospital Plan were kept reasonably accurate by advances in psychiatry which followed it, one may perhaps reasonably hope for advances in the treatment of schizophrenia which will further reduce the institutional needs for this disorder though the warnings of Wing (8) and Baldwin (12) must be heeded. On the other hand, I see no such prospect for dementia and therefore no likelihood of any reduction in bed occupancy there. At the other end of the age range there seems to be a need for expansion in the provision for residential and day treatment of disturbed children and adolescents.

Returning to the question of the mental hospitals, there are certainly important problems over the next few years. The move of the acute units to the DGH is likely to damage morale and to hinder the replacement of existing nursing staff even if it does not actually deplete them. There will also be much insecurity as the number of patients is eventually run down. It is easy to envisage the latter event being delayed for some time by the continued use of beds for psycho-geriatric patients, though this is a situation which one would not wish to prolong, as the elderly are a group who really have strong claims to be admitted to hospital as near to their homes (and thus friends and relations) as possible. One is hopeful therefore that this interregnum will not last too long and that patients will find themselves rehoused in purpose-built and reasonably located accommodation. As I indicated, however, this will be a very traumatic period for the staff and one in which attention to standards of care will need to be very careful indeed.

The therapeutic advances I have mentioned have helped to shorten the functional psychoses, to break them up into discrete episodes or to render them compatible with life in the community. Further refinements have facilitated this, thus the depot phenothiazines may overcome the ambivalence or forgetfulness of the chronic schizophrenic about his medication, and undoubtedly represent a major advance in the long-term care of this disorder. Lithium has proved its prophylactic value, and we may still see an extension of the range of affective disorders to which it can be applied. We might more readily have foregone the explosion of anxiolytic and sedative drugs, which must also have contributed to the epidemic of attempted suicide of the last few years. One might reasonably expect major advances in the field of chemotherapy in the next couple of decades. Less toxic neuroleptics and antidepressants, quicker-acting antidepressants, possible refinement of the chemical alternatives to ECT, and the spread of the depot preparation to the management of affective disorders (and possibly alcoholism and sexual disorders, where progress has already been made) would all pay dividends. It may well be that the precision of our chemotherapy, and our certainty of its administration, will be increased by the spread of serum-level estimations to general rather than just research usage.

Psychiatrists have tended to become increasingly psychodynamic in their outlook and practice, though much less in this country than in USA. The various schools of psycho-analysis still haggle over points of doctrine, but the practising psychiatrist is still likely to use a little of each to provide a framework for group and individual psychotherapy. The importance of group dynamics has also been emphasized in the mushrooming of the 'therapeutic community' which increasingly forms the model, though often much diluted, for many hospital units. Estimates have been made of the potential demand for psychotherapy (8), using conservative criteria, which have indicated that a considerable expansion of this aspect of the service may be needed. Unfortunately attempts to confirm the value of such therapy have either been abandoned because of the methodological constraints or have been of dubious validity. While recognizing that psychotherapeutic skills are necessary for most personnel in the psychiatric field, it would be desirable to have clearer evidence of the specific aspects of these techniques which are of value and exactly which sort of patient is most likely to benefit, before committing ourselves to a major expansion of this service. For we seem to be passing into an era of the fixed budget, and there will be many rival claims.

By contrast there has been more objective evidence of success in the field of behaviour therapy. Based on learning theory and predominantly developed by psychologists the approach is more pragmatic with a concern more for the inconvenience to the patient of his symptoms than their symbolic significance. Manifestations of anxiety have been the most fruitful target of the behaviour therapist, but aversive techniques have had some success in the management of certain sexual deviations and, to a lesser extent, of alcoholism and smoking. There is undoubtedly a wide potential clientele for these therapies and one therefore welcomes the trend towards their refinement and economical administration. Another contribution from experimental psychology has been the application of operant conditioning techniques to the management of behaviour disorders, and the development of training programmes in the field of mental handicap. Most impressive results have been reported and one foresees the extension of this approach into other areas of psychiatry, where techniques of patient care may come to be drastically reviewed (26). Both these areas of advance, as I have mentioned, have been pioneered by psychologists, who have also demonstrated the practicability of training nursing and other staff to carry out the day-to-day administration of the regimes. In the field of behaviour modification this organization of staff attitudes and techniques is fundamental to the success of the programme. For these reasons we must recognize the claims of the clinical psychologist to a position of greater authority within the psychiatric team.

I should also like to consider the changes that have been occurring at the interface between psychiatry and the rest of medicine. The most vital has probably been the recognition of the importance of psychological stress as a precipitant or a complicating factor in physical illness. With the move of psychiatrists into the general hospital this will demonstrate itself in an increasing frequency of requests for advice from the psychiatrist. Such links are particularly desirable with the gynaecologist, the gastro-enterologist, and the neurologist. Now that psychosomatic medicine is less out on a limb and has modified its emphasis to the 'psychosomatic approach' (rather than trying to offer purely psychodynamic explanations for such disorders as asthma and ulcerative colitis), the psychiatrist is likely to be taken more seriously by these specialists, though his grasp of medicine must be better than it generally is now if he is to assess fully the contributions of emotional factors to the patient's condition. In passing one might mention the developing field of biofeedback (again emanating from the psychologist) where operant techniques may eventually prove applicable to the treatment of such common disorders as headaches, peptic ulcer, irritable colon, and even hypertension.

There has fortunately been a marked improvement in the teaching of psychiatry to medical students, and in some places the behavioural sciences are joining their biological counterparts in the early stages of the curriculum. Such a process is being extended into postgraduate education, with senior hospital officer (SHO) rotations into psychiatry proving popular and with a strong psychiatric flavour being added to the training of GPs. The latter, of course, is crucial as one foresees the GP playing a central role in the psychiatric services of the future. Again the presence of the psychiatrist in the general hospital should ensure that he will play an active role in the postgraduate centre and particularly in refresher courses (as teacher and student). Another role for the psychiatrist in the general hospital has been that pioneered at University College Hospital where individual psychiatrists have close links with particular medical teams. Though this may be difficult to achieve in the average district general hospital, it is no doubt a valuable model for the teaching hospital, where the students may be made more aware of the stresses of hospital care to the patient which we all know to be so easily ignored.

Having spoken of the contribution psychiatry might make to other specialties it is relevant to mention the reciprocal. There is a growing literature on the scope of neurosurgery in the treatment of chronic tension and depressive states and of some behaviour disorders. The refinement of frontal leucotomy has made this a much less hazardous procedure than previously and one foresees a continued place for such operations. The ablation of other parts of the limbic system has also been claimed to have effects on mood and tension levels, and particularly on repeated aggressive behaviour. This field, and its ethical ramifications, obviously need careful exploration, though it is unlikely that amygdalectomy will achieve a premature vogue like leucotomy in the 1940s, especially as one recalls the recent promise of behavioural approaches to obsessional neurosis and aggression.

Looking to psychiatric research one hopes that the next couple of decades will shed some light on the confusing issues of aetiology, classification, and biochemistry of the major psychiatric illnesses. We have some idea of the scope of genetic factors, but as yet little about the mechanisms by which they work: thus prophylactic measures seem a long way off, and the application of eugenics unlikely. The role of stress has received more objective confirmation and, with Cooper (15), I shall welcome the day when the social psychiatrist can begin to throw real weight into campaigns to reduce the many environmental stresses which our society continues to create for itself. Conversely, the confident statements from certain schools as to the influence of family dynamics and methods of communication as specific pathogens in the causation of such disorders as schizophrenia seem likely to be undermined as research techniques improve.

The validity of so much research in psychiatry is still limited by our uncertainty in the field of classification. There is still a lot of sterile debate on this topic, but one hopes that the more widespread use of a standardized classification and the use in research of tools which are less bound to traditional disease categories are likely to ensure that future studies, whether by social psychiatrist, biochemist, or psychologist, are more likely to be based on homogenous populations. This would be facilitated by any development of biochemical markers for the particular disorders which, with further therapeutic advances, may arise as by-products of studies of chemical mechanisms. The latter seems a long way off at present, but one is encouraged by a more disciplined approach in some quarters of the research world, the prospective and the controlled study becoming much more the norm. This self-discipline might be carried further, however, in a greater readiness to co-ordinate research towards longer-term goals such as characterizes the work of Wing and his colleagues in the MRC Social Psychiatry Research Unit at Camberwell, and to mount cohort studies from which normative data can be collected. The latter trend might advance further if it was not so widely felt, in psychiatry as in medicine, that a bit of research is good for the young doctor's soul, not to mention his promotion, which undoubtedly fosters a lot of the indifferent or unimportant research which pads out some of our journals.

I have mentioned here the contribution psychiatrists will have to make in exerting social and political pressure to remedy social ills for which they have convincing evidence of guilt. Psychiatrists will probably also be asked to add their comments to those of sociologists, anthropologists, ethologists, and psychologists on other more philosophical problems increasingly bothering our society. With the popularization of scientific knowledge about ourselves and our environment, and with the erosion of the traditional religious and superstitious explanations for the anomalies and hardships of life, the spread of nihilism seems bound to increase. The loss of social hierarchy (and with it the support to the individual of his group identity) and the devaluation of middle and old age, seem likely to add further to these stresses; thus the individual will be exposed to a society of increasing 'anomie', stripped of many of the blinkers to reality which previously enabled him to press on purposefully through adversity. An atheistic psychiatrist already experiences this difficulty in talking to the young 'drop-out' or the older would-be suicide; I think that we shall have this sort of problem on a much wider scale in the future and that the answers will be very difficult to produce. I have often felt that the continued popularity of psycho-analytical concepts among psychiatrists relates to their potential as a humanizing antidote to the determinism of learning theory, and it may be that this will be a potent factor in their survival.

To conclude this section, I would emphasize the continuing migration of the psychiatrist towards the community, which is bound to increase his awareness of the size of some of the icebergs whose tips he has encountered already. I would envisage a further reduction of long-term hospital care as a feature of psychiatry of all but the elderly, and would anticipate that therapeutic advances will once again be on the side of the DHSS prophets. There will be important interim problems for the mental hospitals, whose morale and staffing will suffer, and whose survival may well be extended by financial barriers to purpose-building of units to replace them. The move to the DGH will serve as a challenge to the psychiatrist to share skills and training with his medical colleagues, a theme I shall pursue later on. Just as he may thus revert to a more strictly medical role, the expansion to be expected in the activities of the psychologist points to the latter playing a far more important part in the team in the future, I have also pointed out the responsibility of psychiatrists to co-ordinate their research, to broadcast their socially important findings, and to be prepared (by which I mean equipped) to comment on social dilemmas in the future.

The case-load, and ways of meeting it

I have already pointed out the great reduction in pressure on hospital beds from the functional psychoses; this does not automatically imply a concomitant easing of the workload of the psychiatrist since the incidence of these conditions remains as high. The range of chemotherapy has, however, brought more of these disorders within the scope of the GP. Epidemiologists have indicated the volume of neuroses seen, if not recognized, by the GP (24) and the fact that his choice of cases for specialist referral may not always be appropriate (22). How much of this population should psychiatry tackle? We know how much social disability may arise from chronic neuroses, and claims have been made for the value of psychological intervention in the more acute episode. I have mentioned the promising role of behaviour therapy in the management of disorders in which anxiety is a major symptom, and it is clearly important that those who might benefit should be brought into contact with the specialist service as early as possible. Such an ideal will require greater sophistication at the GP level, easy communication between him and the specialist, and a considerable expansion in psychologist manpower.

NEUROSIS AND PERSONALITY DISORDER

In the case of the acute neuroses the promotion of appropriate intervention by doctor and social worker at the primary care level would seem the best solution (ie the psychiatrist's role will be one of educating his colleagues in handling such cases effectively). In the more chronic and handicapping disorders, however, the specialist service will have to offer more and will have to decide which of its therapeutic methods offers the best mix of economy and long-term benefit, and which specialist should administer the treatment. In costing such proposals it must, of course, be recalled how expensive to the community these chronic neuroses are, not to mention the volume of distress they represent.

The next field in which the psychiatrist has hardly scratched the surface is that of personality disorder. We recognize its importance and its contribution to a wide range of psychiatric and social problems (for example, psychiatric breakdown in the individual or his close relative, delinquency, suicidal attempts, marital disharmony and violence to wife or children, behaviour problems in the children, alcohol and drug abuse, and employment problems—a most costly list in terms of suffering and of demand on the health and social services). Here one deals with people who are often unready to accept psychiatric help, and this poses one of psychiatry's great dilemmas. We have been ready to impose treatment in the past on those whose psychiatric state impairs their judgement of their need of it, even when our range of treatment was pretty limited. Our respect for the liberty of the individual has, however, held us back in the case of the disordered personality unless he has done something very striking, usually invoking pressures from the courts for psychiatric intervention. In my view this whole issue needs careful re-examination in terms of the suffering that is often borne by the spouse and children of such individuals. Obviously if psychiatry were to seek for more authority to act in this field (and I recognize that many would not wish for this) it must increase its likelihood of improving the situation by its intervention, and it must be seen clearly to represent a therapeutic rather than a punitive attitude. It must also, of course, avoid even an appearance of acting for the State. This dilemma also faces the social work profession and indeed one would envisage very close collaboration between the health and social services if more effective means were introduced to deal with this major problem of our society.

If it were accepted that psychiatry was to extend its concern with the problem of personality disorder it would be undertaking a vast new load. The central figure here is likely to be the forensic psychiatrist, whose ranks have expanded rapidly in the last few years. The forensic psychiatrist, usually appointed on a regional level at present, has the advantage of a foot in both health and Home Office services. One might envisage his building up a service for more severe personality disorders based on local centres from which domiciliary support could be given, regional units for 'retraining' and treating those with more severe disturbances or crises, and a national network of secure units such as Grendon Underwood and Broadmoor. Such a service would require close collaboration between the forensic psychiatrist and the general psychiatric and social services on the one hand, and the prison medical and probation services on the other. One would envisage that this widening of the forensic psychiatrist's scope would necessitate the creation of posts on an area rather than just a regional level.

At the local level the forensic psychiatrist would work closely with social workers, probation officers, voluntary organizations, the courts, and his fellow-specialists in child and general psychiatry. The focus of this local service might be a centre to which the client could turn (or be brought) for social, medical, legal, occupational, or financial help, the various professionals concerned providing a consultative service (19). One would envisage this centre coming under the aegis of the social services department and not being based with the other psychiatric services in the hospital. It would also offer support to, and encourage the development of, hostels, lodging panels, club activities, and the like. Its services would be available to both offenders and non-offenders, and it would have an important task in disseminating information and attitudes to the community as a whole. Such a centre might usefully contribute to the management of juvenile behaviour problems, in which one would envisage the forensic psychiatrist playing an important role. He would not, of course, be able to cope with all problems of personality disorder in adult and child psychiatry, but would be responsible for the development of the services, and particularly for their prevention aspects.

At the regional level one would envisage a residential unit not aiming at 'high' security, some of whose clientele would have been referred through the courts. The emphasis would again be on personality disorder and its treatment, as the psychiatrically ill offender requiring treatment of his 'illness', rather than his 'behaviour', would be treated either in the mental hospital or prison. The basis of treatment would be the therapeutic community, using the term in the broadest sense. Because of our uncertainty as to the efficacy of the different milieux which have been proposed for this sort of care, there would be a responsibility on the specialty of forensic psychiatry to vary the nature of these units between regions and to evaluate their results. The sort of answers that are required are as to the relative merits of the group dominated and the authoritarian regime, as to the place of individual and group psychotherapy, and as to the efficacy of behaviour modification in this particular field. These units would be funded on a regional level but would obviously need to retain close links with the areas whence the patients were referred. This would particularly apply in the question of follow-up which has almost invariably been the ingredient lacking in otherwise promising schemes for the treatment of the psychopath.

It cannot be pretended that these regional units could, at an economical cost, achieve the level of security necessary to house the really dangerous individual, a point made repeatedly by Scott (23). There will therefore remain an important place for the special hospitals and for an extension of therapeutic innovations within the prison service, such as Grendon Underwood. The clear need for the latter points to the urgency of the exploitation of the opportunities for social and psychological treatment within the penal system, and for the training of prison staff in remedial as well as custodial skills. The forensic psychiatrist might contribute to this trend by encouraging his colleagues in the prison medical service to extend their contacts with their patients out into the regional and district services I have described. This might be further facilitated by the amalgamation of the prison medical service with the NHS, the most crucial result of which would be the opportunity for deployment of clinical psychologists into the prisons, where their influence could be extensive. Even without such amalgamation it is vital that any therapeutic advances made in the prison setting should not be sacrificed because of the inadequacy of follow-up and inflexibility of discharge procedure which are such bugbears at present.

ALCOHOLISM AND DRUG ABUSE

The dilemmas of psychiatry in relation to alcoholism and drug abuse are similar to those I described under the question of personality disorder, and though the medical model is more easily fitted to them their management ultimately boils down to the same thing. For alcoholism particularly we have much information on the extent and chronicity of the problems, but the psychiatrist's involvement with them has been patchy and generally slight. This is a disorder which warrants early recognition, the difficulty of which has been indicated recently by Griffith Edwards and his colleagues (17). The main focus of help needs to be in the community and in some areas the Councils on Alcoholism have begun to develop this. One might envisage a similar model of service to that proposed for the 'forensic' field with a multidisciplinary local centre and more specialized in-patient units (in this case at an area or district level, according to the demand). These units would generally constitute annexes of the DGH psychiatric unit and might reasonably cope with the acute as well as the rehabilitation aspects of withdrawal. The running of such units would rest with a general psychiatrist with a special interest in alcoholism. As well as systematizing the service in this way (and the DHSS has expressed a willingness to support the expansion of such units) it is most important that the recognition of new cases and their absorption by the service should be facilitated by educating those in a position to spot such cases (social workers, GPs, courts) and promoting a more positive attitude towards their referral for treatment.

The problems of drug abuse are more complicated in view of the greater subcultural element. The role of the doctor in this field seems less clear-cut than for alcoholism, though he must have some involvement. The model set up in the MRC study of drug abuse at Chichester (10) suggests that the organization needs to have much wider links (with the police, schoolteachers, and the like) and that early recognition and social rehabilitation may be much more important than the setting up of formal units. One foresees, however, the continued value of the Phoenix House type of unit for the more established abuser. It would seem more appropriate in future for a psychiatrist with a particular interest in adolescence to fill the medical niche in this team.

CHILD PSYCHIATRY

We have just come to the end of the era of the child guidance clinic as a local education authority service. Although its influence has been an important one, particularly since the child psychiatrist has come to examine some of his premises more carefully, anxiety has been expressed as to whether the service has really been missing large sections of its potential clientele, and whether those processed by it have fared significantly better than the remainder (25). Waiting-lists have often been discouragingly long; a major problem has been the difficulty in getting to grips with the reluctant parent; the in-patient services for the severely disturbed child and, particularly, adolescents have seemed grossly inadequate. With better resources for day and in-patient care, and earlier spotting of the severely disturbed child, one would hope that we might, in future, have to place less reliance on children's homes, converted approved schools, and Borstals for the treatment of emotionally disturbed (as opposed to 'subculturally delinquent') individuals.

The full integration of the child psychiatrist's work into the NHS may provide him with the opportunity to rationalize his role and the organization of his service. In the first place he should function as a specialist in severe behaviour disturbance and developmental disorders in children, working in close conjunction with the paediatrician, clinical and educational psychologists, and specialist in mental handicap. With these colleagues he would be responsible for the development of treatment facilities for such patients, and for the establishment of an effective screening and information service to facilitate their early identification. The latter might receive its input from neonatal and child health high-risk registers, from GPs, schools, and teachers, and through the identification of problem families by the social services department and the general psychiatrist. From the therapeutic point of view the ground of the psychiatrist here seems likely to be encroached on by the clinical psychologist.

The child psychiatrist would obviously still retain some involvement with the more diffuse clientele which has traditionally filled the child guidance clinics, but I see this more as a screening role, probably with a pre-screening by a social worker with specialized experience in the field of child care. If it was established that the child was showing a 'normal reaction to abnormal home circumstances' the implication would be that ongoing management would rest with the agency appropriate to the family pathology (for example, general psychiatry service, forensic or alcoholism service, marriage guidance council) with the child's surveillance being carried out by the field social worker or the GP. As I mentioned, a specialized social worker, preferably the child care specialist of the field social work team, might be involved in this screening and would thus be in a good position to advise the primary care worker involved. This arrangement would have the added advantage of bringing the child psychiatry service more into liaison with the general psychiatry service, thus promoting a greater emphasis on a 'family' approach to treatment. This applies even more to the adolescent psychiatrist who might be even more closely integrated into the general psychiatric team, looking to its psychotherapist, psychologist, and social worker for much of the work currently straddled by himself.

MENTAL HANDICAP

Moving next to this field I must admit that an almost total lack of experience necessarily limits my right to comment. I have already mentioned the major advances which have taken place in methods of training the mentally handicapped individual, and the research which has gone on into the types of institution for his care. I am placing little emphasis on research into causes of mental handicap because, important though this is, it has always tended to take the medical limelight away from the less exotic but more immediate question of caring for the established disorder. The future organization of the services for the mentally handicapped is in a state of flux, and one may perhaps join speculation (2, 16) on how things might change if a more rational service is to be achieved.

Taking the institutions first, what are the relative needs for hospital and basic residential care? It has been suggested that there should be a unit on the DGH site for the assessment of mentally handicapped children on an in-patient or day-patient basis. It seems likely, too, that there will continue to be a need for longer-stay units for those with more severe physical or behavioural disabilities, which could also provide for short-term stay for crisis or relief purposes. No doubt such units will comprise for the time being the existing subnormality hospitals, though in the future one would hope that each district would have its own purpose-built unit; as it would not have the same need for DGH facilities it would not need to be on that site. Houses and hostels, run on family or other models, could then serve those needing residential but not nursing care. Special schools and training centres would provide the training and day-care for these residents, as well as those still living with their families, and possibly for at least some of those in the hospital units.

With the spread of responsibility for the care of the mentally handicapped to involve education and social services departments as well as the hospital and community health services, and with the increasing importance of the psychologist in the remedial aspects of care, the management structure of the service clearly needs modification. In this the power of the consultant psychiatrist seems bound to be eroded, and at the same time his role (and thus his training) will need to be rationalized within a multidisciplinary framework. What should the medical member of such a team have to offer? He will have to co-ordinate the contribution to the care of the mentally handicapped individual of a wide range of medical specialists. The primary medical care which he has provided in the mental subnormality hospital would shrink in a hostel and home-based service, since patients would retain their own GPs; in the long-stay hospital unit such care might also be provided by a GP, on a sessional basis. In the assessment unit the specialist would liaise closely and share responsibility with the paediatrician and the child psychiatrist. It might be claimed that these latter specialists could, in fact, provide the whole medical service for the handicapped child, but I think that it is crucial to have a specialist involved in the care at that stage who represents longer-term responsibility than those specialists could offer. This individual would also need to collaborate closely with the community physician at both district and area level, and one might envisage his having a role in the former's department. The consultant in mental handicap would therefore need a thorough grounding in medicine, paediatrics, and medical rehabilitation; he would also need training at a registrar level in psychiatry and, particularly, child psychiatry; assuming a greater emphasis in the medical schools on the problems of mental handicap he might be offered this specialist training at such centres.

With the shift to the community the influence of the social worker in the team must increase. There will be a need for someone with sufficient authority within the social services division to co-ordinate the residential provisions, the day-centres, training centres, and other sources of sheltered employment, as well as to advise and influence field social workers dealing with the mentally handicapped and their families. As a member of the team this social worker would have close links with the hospital units, and would play an important part in admission and discharge plans for those units. Like the consultant he would need to liaise closely with the community physician's representative in the field at a district and area level to make sure that their respective resources interlocked adequately.

Another section of the team which would assume increasing importance comprises those concerned with training. One would like to see a senior member of the local education department playing a full role in the team's planning as well as in the administration of the special schooling which is already that department's responsibility. This person would work closely with the psychologist who would assess and set up training programmes for the individual child (or adult). Between them they would develop such programmes in the setting of the special schools, as well as the homes, hostels, and 'hospital' units. The psychologist, who would probably be employed by the health authority, would therefore be involved in the supervision of teachers, residential care staff, and nurses in such programmes, and would thus be an important figure in the service.

Although the nursing administrator in the team might be commanding a diminishing force the influence would be a broader one. Just as doctor and psychologist would have to emerge from the hospital there will be a need for nurses with experience in handling the mentally handicapped to go out into the community to give support and advice to relatives and to the staff of hostels. Senior nurses will also have an important part to play in the training of residential care staff, and one hopes that these trends will lead to a greater awareness in the hospitals of the problems of the community, and vice versa. The same spread between hospital and community will be necessary on the part of other remedial professions such as physiotherapy and occupational therapy. Both nursing staff and remedial therapists would play an important part in the carrying out of training programmes in the hospital setting and maintaining these if the patients leave hospital. The broader, less medical, function of the 'nurse' is bound to have its impact on training.

I have emphasized the replacement of the old hospital-based

autocracy by community-based teamwork. It has been suggested that this should go further, with the development of a unified service for the mentally handicapped autonomous within the field of health and social services with its own national structure. This would certainly facilitate co-ordination of services and enable pressure to be exerted locally and nationally for their improvement. On the other hand it might have an isolating effect on the clientele and on the professionals involved. I feel that the benefits of such a service could be achieved by a specialist team such as I have discussed, with each drawing on the resources of his own larger department or profession, provided that it really does work as a team, bestowing leadership on those who contribute most to its success, rather than on a member of one particular discipline on a basis of divine right.

PSYCHIATRY OF THE ELDERLY

The other major field of psychiatric morbidity to be considered, and again one which psychiatry has tended to neglect, is in the elderly. We are aware of the particular vulnerability of this group, with its high prevalence of both functional and organic disorders, and of the rapid expansion of its ranks, especially among the very aged. Recognition of this load, and the extent to which it has already overtaken the resources of the psychiatric services, have led recently to a rapid expansion of a new subspecialty, psycho-geriatrics. Deviating from the pattern for the psychiatric care proposed for the elderly by successive DHSS circulars (3) some authors, notably Arie (6), have described comprehensive services for the elderly dealing with both functional and organic disorders. The benefits in terms of morale and expertise in a service with the latter approach make it likely that this will become the norm in the future.

The psycho-geriatrician has to link very closely with both geriatric and social services departments to ensure that their related services work to the best advantage; he will also need the goodwill of his general psychiatry colleagues who will obviously still cope with a proportion of the uncomplicated psychiatry of this age-group. As psychiatry moves into the general hospital it becomes easier for psycho-geriatrician and geriatrician to merge administratively. There will be need for joint-user units, more along the lines described by Arie and Dunn (11) than of the generally proposed psycho-geriatric assessment units. I emphasize this because it is clear that a comprehensive psychiatric service for the elderly requires many more acute beds than the norms for these assessment units, while the number of patients for whom joint care and assessment is needed is smaller than those norms (3). The close links I have mentioned would facilitate the training of staff, the exchange of ideas, the service to the individual patient, and the presentation of a combined front for the collaboration with other agencies in the district, and for applying pressure for a better share of the health budget for the elderly.

I have mentioned that psycho-geriatrics has been the one area of expanding chronic bed occupancy in our specialty. The norms recommended by the DHSS (3) seem frighteningly low when one is confronted with overflowing hospitals and considerable numbers of patients constituting risk to themselves or heavy burdens on their families and the community services. Day care and appropriate use of beds may partially remedy this, but it is clear that there will be an increasing need in the future for specialization in residential care to accommodate the mentally infirm, with corresponding support from the psycho-geriatrician. Before leaving the question of in-patient care one must emphasize the importance of maintaining morale and standards in what is potentially the least rewarding area of nursing, the long-stay psycho-geriatric ward. The role of occupational therapists in these areas can be very helpful, and one is anxious to examine the possibilities of operant conditioning and of other methods of facilitating 'learning' with demented patients. The whole emphasis of this sector of care must be on the maintenance of the quality of life (which gradually shifts from participation in the environment to bodily comfort as dementia proceeds) and not on recovery, and certainly not on the prolongation of life.

I have dealt at some length with these more immediate problems, but one looks ahead to much more positive horizons. I have indicated that there must be close liaison with other disciplines dealing with the elderly. The target of the psycho-geriatrician, like the geriatrician, must be to partake in a service which promotes the over-all health and quality of life of the elderly. Such a service will need to involve housing, education, social services, and community health departments, the GPs and the community nursing services (which should include psycho-geriatric nurses liaising with the psycho-geriatricians), and above all the volunteer. It must occupy itself with preparing people for retirement, with schemes to identify and reduce isolation, immobility, and inactivity among the elderly, with clubs, day-centres, libraries, good neighbour schemes, provision of sheltered housing, residential care, and hospital care. Only if all are looked at together will it be appreciated that it is in the field services and housing schemes that the great expansion must take place. The part of the psycho-geriatrician in all of this will, of course, be predominantly indirect, and even in the care of those showing psychiatric morbidity his role will be one of supporting a service with its focus at the primary care level.

PREVENTIVE PSYCHIATRY

Having dealt with some of the areas in which psychiatry is faced with an obvious demand on its services I should like to look beyond these to ways in which a more preventive approach may be possible. I shall not dwell on the possibility of advances in research which may lead to specific prophylaxis for major psychiatric illnesses as I do not see this as more than speculation at present. In a more general sense research may consolidate evidence to attribute the onset or exacerbation of such disorders to specific environmental hazards (such as noise, tower blocks, industrial working conditions) or to social underprivilege. As Cooper (15) has recently emphasized it will be the duty of the social psychiatrist and the epidemiologist to draw general attention to such findings and, if necessary, to exert social and political pressure to minimize such risks in the future. This sort of work and, one hopes, some clarification of predisposing factors in delinquency research could begin to enable psychiatry to exert a major influence on the sort of society we create for ourselves, though we must learn the lessons of the past and not go beyond the limits of our evidence.

Prevention is also, of course, an important target in many aspects of the practice of psychiatry today, and was fundamental to the philosophy of child guidance. A recent development, more popular in the USA than this country has been that of crisis intervention. The principle is that people are at their most impressionable in terms of courses of action at the height of their anxiety at a time of stress. If they manage to respond appropriately to the stress their anxiety will fall and they may cope more confidently with other stresses in the future; if they fail to do so they may develop habitually poor patterns of response and the old anxieties will be easily evoked. The implication is that the latter is the pathway to psychiatric illness, though such links have not as yet been demonstrated. The practical model of crisis intervention is that the person under stress searches for help and if he can find someone with insight his response is likely to be more successful. The helper in this situation aims to keep the individual repeatedly facing and attempting to solve his dilemma and, as the process develops successfully, withdraws his support and advice. It is therefore a brief form of therapy but intensive while at its peak. Crisis intervention centres in the USA have staff of various disciplines and may work on an out-patient, day-patient, or in-patient basis, and deal with a wide range of problems extending into the field of psychiatric illness.

One cannot envisage the psychiatric services in this country laying on this sort of service with all its other commitments; it may, however, contribute to such developments through the training of those who professionally or voluntarily find themselves in crisis intervention situations, though there are, of course, many instances when the psychiatrist himself must take this approach with his patients. Others likely to benefit from such training are GPs, social workers, the clergy, members of organizations such as the Samaritans, and personnel officers. One type of crisis in which the psychiatrist is all too often involved these days is that of attempted suicide. These situations provide good models of the crisis situation, with the subject initially choosing a fugitive response to the stress, but it is argued that the period following the overdose (or its equivalent) is still ripe for intervention. A project is planned in Southampton (18) to evaluate such intervention by a social worker (a by-product of which may be the conclusion that the psychiatrist need see far fewer such patients). Wherever other professionals or lay workers are forming the backbone of such a para-psychiatric service it is, of course, crucial that the psychiatric service is ready to back them up by readily seeing anyone whom they feel to be getting out of hand. In this respect every district psychiatric service should be able to offer a real twenty-four hour emergency service for the walk-in variety.

Teamwork in psychiatry

Throughout this paper I have been pointing out areas of expansion for psychiatry. I do not imply by this that a great increase in recruitment of psychiatrists will be necessary and should like now to discuss ways in which the manning of these services might be rationalized. I have already indicated that the icebergs I have mentioned have been tackled in a hitherto rather disjointed way by GPs, social workers, and the community nursing services. It is predominantly at this primary care level that such problems are best handled, and if psychiatry is to advance its practical contribution to society it must be by facilitating this sort of care. In the next few pages I shall consider how these workers might be moulded into an effective primary care team (the model for which has already been established in several centres) and how the specialist service might deploy itself to support such a team.

The organization of primary health care teams, and their relationships to other parts of the health and social services, will be dealt with elsewhere in this book. My theme is simply that with the sort of training which is currently proposed for GPs, social workers, and health visitors, and with access to specialist advice and treatment resources, such a primary care team could cope effectively with the bulk of psychiatric morbidity. I appreciate that it will be a long time before people with adequate training comprise the majority of such teams, and indeed before the necessary integration is satisfactorily achieved, but this should be the goal towards which we are working.

Taking the ideal model of such a team one envisages a group of four to six GPs who would have had some undergraduate teaching in behavioural sciences and psychiatry, and with further psychiatric experience during their postgraduate training. One member might have a particular interest in psychiatry, possibly doing a couple of sessions in this field as a clinical assistant; he would not do the practice's psychiatry but he would be a source of advice for his colleagues and of liaison with the specialist service. These GPs might therefore reasonably be expected to recognize and offer physical treatment or simple psychotherapy to patients whose presentation suggested emotional or psychiatric problems. If further advice was needed they could look to the specialists; if investigation or modification of the family dynamics or social problems was desirable they would refer the matter to the social worker or health visitor, rather than apply palliative medication as tends to be the case at present.

These other workers would either deal with the matter on the basis of their own training and experiences or enlist the support of their own specialist colleagues. (Each field social work team might include an individual with special experience in mental health [as well as others in child care and care of the elderly] to whom they would have easy access, and who would in fact function also as a member of the specialist team, to which we shall come later.) Similarly I anticipate the extension of the present deployment of psychiatric nurses in the community so that each nursing team in the community could have its own psychiatric (and psychogeriatric) specialist who would offer support to his or her 'generic' colleagues as well as having close links with the nursing officer and psychiatrist of the specialist team.

Space does not permit detailed discussion of the feasibility of such teamwork, though examples of its success (14) suggest that it will become more generalized as attitudes change and administrative problems are overcome. For such a team to tackle psychiatric problems effectively the training and support which I have mentioned are essential, and the teething problems of Seebohm and the currently inadequate numbers of social workers should not be regarded as permanent obstacles. I would emphasize that the improvements in psychiatry which I have discussed will depend as much as anything on a considerable increase in the social work establishment. What I see as the great potential strength of this primary care team is that it will function together over a wide range of social and health problems, of which psychiatric disorder will only be one facet; it is less likely therefore to miss the family problems which underlie so much of the latter. It also offers a far better guarantee of continuity of care than the present specialist-based service. Thus it would use the specialist team for advice and the provision of (usually short) spells of treatment, while retaining over-all responsibility in so far as this was feasible.

Passing on to the specialist team, I see this comprising the same disciplines as at present but with marked changes in their relationship to each other, to the primary care team, and to the patient, some of which I shall go on to discuss. I envisage the specialist team serving a population equivalent to about half a dozen average-sized group practices. This would be similar to the scope of the 'team' proposed in the circular, *Services for the Mentally Ill* (1), and in the report of the Tripartite Committee (5), and would mean that there would usually be three or four teams in each district. Both these publications recommended that the team functioned on a multidisciplinary basis, though I should like to see the roles of the constituent professions altered more radically still to ensure that each is working predominantly within the range of his basic training and special expertise.

To consider the psychiatrist first, I see him constricting his role considerably. As the medical specialist in the team he needs to show a far greater proficiency in neurology, general medicine, and clinical pharmacology than is generally the case at present. These are areas in which he is repeatedly asked for advice (or should be) and, with the move to the general hospital and the increasing potency and range of side-effects of medication, this is bound to increase. He will, of course, retain an important role in the diagnosis and treatment of the functional psychoses, but I feel that he will need to loosen his grip on some of the psychological methods of treatment for which he is far less specifically trained. This will mean that his central role of clinical responsibility within the specialist team is likely to be eroded. Many patients referred by the primary care team will be for specialized psychological treatment or casework and will be sent directly to the appropriate specialist. No doubt the psychiatrist will still play an important screening role even in such cases, but the assumption would not be that he will be the one to administer or retain clinical responsibility for the treatment, unless it is specifically a medical one.

Psychiatrists will obviously wish to develop fields of special interest within which they may function as the district 'expert'. This would apply, for instance, to rehabilitation, alcoholism, drug abuse, and sexual problems. It would be desirable that they should take the medical share of the responsibility for specialized services of this sort in the district, and might devote some sessions entirely to such work, but one would still see them functioning as 'generic' psychiatrists within the sub-district specialist team. I do not foresee in the near future the need for further development of discrete subspecialties within psychiatry other than those I have mentioned previously.

By contrast I see a considerable expansion in the workload, clinical responsibility, and establishment of the clinical psychologist. The range of his skills, the number of patients to whom these will be applied, and the extent to which the psychologist will train and delegate nursing staff and other aides in such treatment must establish for him the right to the same sort of autonomy within the specialist team as the doctor. The findings of the Trethowan Committee (4) are likely to promote such a trend, though I feel that the consultative document is too cautious about his independence from doctors. I therefore envisage the psychologist providing a consultant service to the primary care team, to members of the specialist team, and to other medical specialists, and conducting programmes of behaviour therapy and modification in collaboration with his colleagues, both in and outside the hospital setting. There is bound to be specialization within the distinct psychology service, but one hopes that the 'specialist team' I have been considering would include a psychologist of fairly broad skills.

I have already mentioned that I anticipate each social service fieldwork team having its specialist in mental health, and that this individual would be a member of the psychiatric specialist team. As well as offering guidance and training to field social workers I see this individual having an important part to play in the organization of care in the hospital setting, and in the provision of psychotherapy. Again, this specialist social worker would function as an autonomous consultant within the team, and would, for instance, need to be able to admit patients to hospital on his own discretion. One hopes that this incorporation of a member of the social services department in the specialist team would further foster relations between the two services, and pave the way to their possible future amalgamation.

So far in this paper I have been lukewarm on the topic of psychotherapy. I doubt the specificity of some of the benefits attributed to its more intensive regimes, and certainly see little place for the latter in a service with such a large clientele. It will, however, be necessary to train and supervise workers in techniques of psychotherapy, especially of the group and supportive variety. In many instances this might be done by the psychiatric social worker (PSW), but it seems likely that each district should have a full-time psychotherapist, who would give sessions to each specialist team for this purpose, as well as having patients in treatment himself, and supervising any specialized 'therapeutic community' developed in the district. Various authors (7) and bodies (9) have emphasized the need to train such specialists, though there has been debate as to whence they should be recruited. One hopes that the trend will be towards more non-medical psychotherapists, as it seems both uneconomical and illogical to prefix such a career with a medical training which is irrelevant and often antipathetic to it. Along with such a trend the psychotherapist would widen his sphere of influence well beyond the established health professions, by giving support to such agencies as Samaritans, Marriage Guidance Councils, and the clergy. His role as a teacher would be quite as important as his actual involvement in therapy.

I shall not go into details on the role of the nursing officer and the remedial therapist in the specialist team except to emphasize the greater flexibility that would be required from their staff in the future, and thus the greater responsibility they would have in maintaining the therapeutic milieu and staff morale. Both would also need to strengthen their links with the community services (the nursing officer through an advisory role *vis-à-vis* the community psychiatric nurses, and the occupational therapist through greater contact with her opposite numbers in the social services department, and in the services for the mentally and physically handicapped and the elderly). It has also to be emphasized that until the NHS starts paying its occupational therapists a respectable wage it will continue to deserve to have even more unfilled posts than it has at present.

The rather specialized field of psychiatric rehabilitation would probably best be organized on a district basis, with leadership shared by a clinical psychologist, an occupational therapist, and a psychiatrist. The former two individuals would probably work outside the specialist team structure while the psychiatrist might be a member of one of the teams with a particular interest, giving some sessions to the rehabilitation unit. They would be responsible for the over-all standard of the service, as well as for liaison with equivalent services in the community and with the medical rehabilitation service. It seems certain that the problems of rehabilitation and the maintenance of a positive attitude to the treatment of patients with chronic disability will remain important aspects of the district psychiatric service long after the existing backlog has been dealt with.

This leads me finally to consider the interaction of this team with other parts of the service. I have discussed the need for easy communication between members of the specialist team and between them and the primary team. Each member of the primary care team has a member of his own profession in the specialist team and these will probably form the strongest links. For the whole system to run smoothly it is obviously crucial that the specialist team, catering as it would be for about 60,000 people, has the same catchment area as the equivalent sub-team of the social services division. It should not be impossible for both to organize their boundaries along practice divisions (rather as health visitor teams often do already) particularly if the GPs in their turn attempt to round off the geographical spread of their caseload. The latter trend would, of course, be greatly facilitated by the health centre system, not to mention the arrival of a salaried GP service.

The specialist team would be strengthened by the partial involvement, as I have outlined already, of the various other psychiatric specialists (child psychiatrist, adolescent psychiatrist, forensic psychiatrist); in turn individual psychiatrists in each district would co-ordinate the medical aspects of the rehabilitation, alcoholism, and drug abuse services. The overlap with the specialists in mental handicap and psychiatry for the elderly would be slight, as each would be involved with their separate district services. Another area of liaison on which I should have placed more emphasis is that with the district community physician, fortified probably by a specialist community physician from the area. The health care planning team would need to incorporate adequate representation of this wide range of disciplines concerned with the psychiatric service, and would need to move closely in step with the 'district' director of social services and the area officers involved in his planning. The psychiatrists would obviously retain their own professional links at a district and regional level, as well as through their Royal College, and no district medical committee would be complete without a psychiatrist. Similarly, the psychologists would have their separate organization, and one trusts that at district, area, regional, and national level their representation in psychiatric planning would be encouraged by the psychiatrists. There would still be a need at district level, however, for a multidisciplinary equivalent to the Cogwheel division, and it would be desirable for the psychiatrist on the district medical committee to be elected from this group, rather than his psychiatric colleagues alone.

Conclusion

In this paper I have outlined some of the major changes in emphasis which I would anticipate in the psychiatric services in the next couple of decades. The move to the DGH is, of course, well under way and with it the opportunity to make better use of day-care and to offer a flexible use of hospital facilities that was less possible with the geographical separation of the mental hospital from its base population. The latter institution will obviously be with us for a long time yet, but the next few years, with the probable bonus of further therapeutic advances, should give the opportunity to assess whether additional community supports and development of smaller specialized units will adequately supplement the DGH facilities in a comprehensive service.

I have gone on to consider other responsibilities which I feel that psychiatry will have to tackle more systematically than at present. If it is to do so it will either have to engage in a massive expansion of the specialist service, which would not be viable, or to equip the fieldworkers of the health and social services to cope with the load, backed by a more streamlined specialist service. The cornerstone of such a system would be the primary care team of GP, social worker, and community nurse. If current trends in the training of these professions is enhanced by a more purposeful contribution from psychiatry, and if the specialist service is organized in a way which promotes easy access and support (but without the takeover of care which characterizes the service at present), this primary team should be well placed to provide the sort of care necessary and to tie it in with other services to each family concerned. One important proviso, however, is that there should be a considerable expansion in numbers of social workers in the area teams, and that they and the GPs are prepared to be swayed by the experience of those who have found this sort of teamwork valuable, and thus to break down inter-professional barriers.

In my consideration of the specialist team and its relations with other disciplines I have emphasized the need for a much more careful review of the individual professional roles than has been generally accepted. The psychiatrist should function more effectively as a medical opinion within the team and for his GP and hospital specialist colleagues. He should no longer be the central figure of clinical responsibility in the psychiatric team, and should withdraw from any major role in the psychological methods of treatment. I would therefore see it as unlikely that the establishment of psychiatrists will need to increase. By contrast the breadth and depth of the clinical psychologist's responsibilities seem bound to increase, and, with this, his establishment and autonomy within the team. One hopes that the recognition of this fact which is bound to follow the Trethowan Committee's report will make recruitment easier than it has been under the existing cramped conditions. I have also favoured the development of a separate specialty of psychotherapy with a sphere of activity extending well outside the NHS (by which I do not mean the private sector) and with its recruitment generally from outside the medical profession. I have also emphasized the role of the 'psychiatric' social worker, linking the specialist team with its equivalent social service team, but also playing an important executive and advisory role in both directions. I would regard this sort of specialist (along with others in child care and care of the elderly) as crucial to the survival of generic social work teams, and to liaison with the hospital service. It would also be an important link to have established in the event of health and social services amalgamating, with all the advantages that this might bring to psychiatry.

I am aware of the massive assumptions and snags inherent in these proposals. As I indicated at the beginning of the paper I have slanted my comments towards a personal viewpoint and away from passive or objective prophecy. In defence of this, however, I would say that I can see no way in which a psychiatric service of the size that the suffering in our society warrants could be provided by a specialist-orientated system such as we have at present. I feel therefore that our first priority must be to work out how the generalists can be helped to provide it themselves, and this must be backed by greater readiness on the part of psychiatrists to rationalize their own function within the service.

I should like to acknowledge my gratitude to my secretary, Mrs Hazel Draper, who despite a heavy workload and domestic commitments has found the time to type the drafts of this paper. I apologise to those whose ideas I have cannibalized without so much as a reference, or with reference only to a publication in which they were one among many contributors.

REFERENCES

1. Department of Health and Social Security (1971). *Hospital Services for the Mentally Ill*, HM (71) 79 (London: HMSO).
2. —— (1971). *Better Services for the Mentally Handicapped.* Cmnd. 4683 (London: HMSO).
3. —— (1972). *Services for Mental Illness Related to Old Age*, HM (72) 71 (London: HMSO).
4. —— (1974). Consultative Document (on the role of the clinical psychologist).
5. British Medical Association Tripartite Committee (1972). *The Mental Health Services after Reunification.*
6. McLachlan, G. (ed.) (1972). *Approaches to Action.* Occasional Hundreds 5 (Oxford University Press for the Nuffield Provincial Hospitals Trust).
7. Cawley, R., and McLachlan, G. (eds) (1973). *Policy for Action* (Oxford University Press for the Nuffield Provincial Hospitals Trust).
8. Wing, J. K., and Hailey, A. M. (1972). *Evaluating a Community Psychiatric Service* (Oxford University Press for the Nuffield Provincial Hospitals Trust).
9. *Psychotherapy—Do we need more 'Talking Treatment'?* (1974). Mind Report no. 12 (London: NAMH).
10. de Alarcon, R. (1971). World Congress of Psychiatry, Mexico (to be published in the Proceedings).
11. Arie, Tom, and Dunn, Tom (1973). *Lancet*, ii, 1313.
12. Baldwin, J. A. (1971). *The Mental Hospital in the Psychiatric Services* (Oxford University Press for the Nuffield Provincial Hospitals Trust).
13. Brothwood, J. (1971). In Kay, D. W. K., and Walk, A. (eds). *Recent Developments in Psychogeriatrics* (RMPA).
14. Cooper, B. (1971). *Lancet*, i, 539.
15. —— (1973). *Psychol. Med.* 3, 401.

16. DAY, K. (1974). *Br. J. Psychiat. Suppl.* (April), 13.
17. EDWARDS, G., *et al.* (1973). *Br. J. Psychiat.* 123, 169.
18. GIBBONS, J. L. (1973). Personal communication.
19. GUNN, JOHN (1971). *Br. J. Hosp. Med.* 6, 260.
20. HILL, DENIS (1969). *Psychiatry in Medicine*, Rock Carling Monograph (London: Nuffield Provincial Hospitals Trust).
21. MANN, S. A. (1974). *Spring Quarterly Meeting of the Royal College of Psychiatrists.*
22. RAWNSLEY, K., and LOUDON, J. B. (1962). *Br. J. prev. soc. Med.* 16, 174.
23. SCOTT, P. D. (1974). Spring Quarterly Meeting of Royal College of Psychiatrists.
24. SHEPHERD, M. *et al.* (1966). *Psychiatric Illness in General Practice* (London: Oxford University Press).
25. —— *et al.* (1971). *Childhood Behaviour and Mental Health* (ULP).
26. TENNANT, T. G., and MARSHALL, J. R. (1974). *Br. J. Hosp. Med.* 11, 89.

A pattern for surgery

JEAN TURNER

JEAN TURNER
MB, ChB, FRCSEd, FRCS
General surgeon

A pattern for surgery

Does general surgery exist? Can general surgery survive? Is there a need still for the general surgeon? Are surgeons increasingly becoming unthinking technical experts? Many are the doubts and the questionings about the future of the major specialty of surgery in our Health Service, and especially of the man who now calls himself a general surgeon. Those of us who remain firmly convinced of the value, present and future, of the skills now embodied in general surgery and of those who execute those skills must find logical arguments to justify that conviction to the sceptics and the cynics.

What then *is* general surgery? Its existence is proved daily in hundreds of NHS general hospitals throughout the length and breadth of the land, where individual surgeons are working their way through operating lists which range from thyroidectomies and gastrectomies to haemorrhoidectomies and Zadik procedures. Of course a different specialist *could* be found for each of these (one who might, through much practice, use a marginally better technique or a different procedure), but is there any real need? The general surgeon has sufficient experience and practice to ensure that he performs these common operations safely and satisfactorily, and in order to take over all such cases, specialist surgeons would have to be many more in number, thereby reducing the value of their concentration on one specialty, as their experience with rarer cases was diluted. Furthermore, the GP could hardly refer every surgical case directly to a specialist surgeon; this would imply home investigation to a level beyond the scope of most general practices in order to select the appropriate specialist. General surgery must therefore survive, and its exponents cannot be expected to be mere 'middlemen' for diagnosis and further referral of patients.

Those who consider that surgeons are approaching the status of mere adept technicians would do well to cast a glance backwards in time, to the barber surgeons who were precisely that: they were skilful in excising visible swellings or opening obvious abscesses. Since those early days, progress has been consistently away from purely technical skills, first as surgery was brought firmly within the profession of medicine, and later as medicine came further within the ambit of science. There remain simple technical cases in which the diagnosis and the treatment are obvious, but there are many others where scientific methods and the combined art and science of clinical judgement are extensively used in investigation, treatment, and post-operative care, and it is precisely this mixture of the intellectual and the practical which appeals to the type of person who chooses surgery as a profession: the man who is a clinical doctor at heart, and a highly trained physician and scientist in intellect, and who *in addition* finds satisfaction in the dexterous use of his hands. Indeed in some fields, particularly those most highly specialized, the borders between medical and surgical specialists are now very much blurred, and the current trend towards discussion between disciplines, both in the abstract and over the particular clinical case, must surely continue.

It has been said that the tendency to increasing subdivision, or 'super-specialization', in surgery is incompatible with the continuance of general surgery. Is this so? Let us consider the present situation in Britain with its National Health Service, and a possible national 'pattern' for surgical practice in the future.

There are today five different types of surgeon. At the centre of everything, the general surgeon works on a varied group of cases, mainly in the DGH; his patients are referred directly to him by a GP or a non-surgical colleague, and in the majority he deals with the problem and returns the patient to his home; he may select a minority to send to a more specialized colleague elsewhere. The specialist surgeon, for example the neurosurgeon, orthopaedic surgeon, or cardiothoracic surgeon, *may* also practise in a district general hospital but is more likely to be found in a regional centre for his specialty; his patients generally belong fairly obviously in his field, and are referred to him also by GPs, physicians, or other colleagues. Thirdly, there is the general surgeon with a special interest in a particular field, such as urology, gastro-enterology, or endocrinology: most general surgeons in university hospitals are of this type, and many in DGHs have developed skills of a similar nature through a sustained interest, known to their colleagues, in such topics. The distinction between these special interests and the major surgical specialties of the previous group is that the bulk of these 'special interest' cases *could* be dealt with by any competent general surgeon (prostatectomies do not have to be in the hands of a urologist) whereas few general surgeons would wish to tackle a pulmonary lobectomy or remove a cerebellar tumour when an appropriate specialist was available. The fourth category embodies the 'super-specialists': those who practise *exclusively* in a limited field such as those special interests already cited, or perhaps yet more exclusively, for example in hepatology, proctology, or paediatric cardiac surgery. These men practise chiefly in what are becoming known as 'centres of excellence', in their own highly specialized units, most of their patients being referred secondarily by hospital colleagues after some investigation. At the opposite pole is the final group: those who practise surgery at its most general, and who are indeed prepared to tackle thoracotomies and craniotomies, gynaecology, orthopaedics, and plastic surgery, simply because they are in situations where it may be necessary for them to do so. Most of these are in developing areas overseas, but a few remain in remote and far-flung parts of our land.

Are all these different surgeons necessary, or must we begin to make choices? Can they all be reconciled with the future NHS in the United Kingdom? I believe that they can, and should: but in a planned arrangement, and with a system of referral of patients, to one category or from one category to another, which is considerably less haphazard than at present. A pattern must be found which will retain the benefits brought by each type of surgeon to society, while at the same time preserving the great NHS ideal of free and equal availability of the optimum treatment for his condition to every sufferer.

Since the rational way to seek a safe formula for any scheme in medicine is to start from the needs of the patient, let us begin by considering the present and future possibilities for a mythical 'Mr A'.

Mr A attends his GP, complaining of dyspepsia. The history is short, the patient fairly young; the practitioner prescribes a simple antacid and a bland diet, and asks Mr A to report back if the condition does not resolve rapidly. A week later Mr A returns, still with 'indigestion' and now also mentioning some epigastric pain, which is relieved temporarily by the antacid. Finding nothing abnormal on examination, the doctor recommends a week of rest at home and regular doses of antacid, in addition to diet. Despite this, the pain persists and increases, and on the next examination the GP finds marked epigastric tenderness. At this point Mr A is referred to the lynch-pin of our present and future surgical service: the general surgeon in his local district general hospital. The GP may or may not have had facilities for barium meal X-ray, but in any case this is done and confirms his diagnosis of an active duodenal ulcer . . . not responding to his treatment.

Let us then suppose that the general surgeon, on pursuing his routine investigations, finds a level of gastric hypersecretion which is virtually diagnostic of the rare Zollinger-Ellison syndrome. Three courses of action are open to him: (1) he may continue to manage the case himself, although his own particular interest is in urology; (2) he may refer Mr A to a colleague in his own hospital whose interest is in gastro-enterology, and who will take over the case for further investigation and either treatment or further referral; (3) he, or his colleague, may communicate urgently with Professor X, whose almost exclusive interest is in surgical conditions of the pancreas, and as a result recommend to Mr A that he be transferred many miles to the professor's special unit for treatment. (Here it may be noted that Mr A has little choice in the matter: he is not in a position to choose, to reject the recommendation, not only because of his lack of medical knowledge, but because proper treatment for his rare condition is not available in his district or region.) Mr A is transferred, has the best treatment available, and is discharged home, to be followed up at intervals in his own DGH, with advice from Professor X as necessary. If, however, our local surgeon chose to retain Mr A within his own unit or within the region, Mr A, if he recovered (or his family if he did not), would probably never know that he had been at greater risk than was necessary because of less-than-optimum care. Any blame would lie squarely with the surgeon, who presumably *knew* where optimum care lay. If, on the other hand, Mr A flatly refused to accept the advice that he should be transferred far away from his home and family, then the general surgeon would have no option but to treat this rare condition to the best of his ability; our future system must try to ensure that his best will not fall too far short of Professor X's standard.

Alternatively, suppose Mr A's symptoms were found initially to be due to an ordinary uncomplicated duodenal ulcer. What does our general surgeon, with his interest in urology, do now? Of course he can quite justifiably treat such a common condition by the most straightforward, standard methods of his day. On the other hand he may know that his surgical colleague's practice (in our present-day example) is to treat duodenal ulcers by highly selective vagotomy, which he himself is not prepared, equipped, or trained to do. If the patient is a reasonably intelligent person, the choice between the tried-and-proven technique and the newer operation may be discussed with him. Such a common condition is unlikely to be referred to a 'super-specialist' unless perhaps where the appropriate one has his practice in the patient's own district; but either of the above pair of surgeons in the district general hospital can be relied upon to handle it safely and adequately.

If, however, Mr A's persistent epigastric pain proves to be due to a carcinoma of the lower oesophagus which is shown to extend upwards to the aortic arch, the general surgeon (or the GP if the barium meal was ordered by him) would be expected to refer the patient immediately to a specialist thoracic surgeon in the same region, the latter's results being predictably better than those of a general surgeon operating in a field to which he is unaccustomed; again our general surgeon is blameworthy if he does not give the patient this opportunity within the region.

For the sake of argument, imagine, as a fourth possibility, that Mr A's pain is eventually found to be due to a very extensive renal carcinoma. Our original surgeon, although interested in urology, wishes to give his patient the best possible chance, and therefore consults with Professor Y in another far-off centre of excellence. But (*a*) Professor Y's lists for the next few weeks are completely full, not only with difficult reconstructional problems, but with fairly routine calculi, bladder tumours, and even prostates which have filtered through to him; and (*b*) Mr A would much prefer to be treated near to his home and family. In a condition which, while not everyday, is far from rare, surely the solution would be if our surgeon, already interested in urology, could be confident that his results did not differ significantly from those of the super-specialist urologist.

Herein lies one possibility for improving the service; although much of the present system works well for many patients, we can at this point embark on our streamlining, with a view to standardizing the service for all. Professor Y *ought* not to be overloaded with cases which are neither rare nor exceptionally difficult; but he has been compelled to offer to operate on them on requests from surgeons who, while they would have enjoyed the procedure, were reluctant to undertake it lest they should give their patients anything other than the best chance, or be accused of dabbling in what should be the super-specialist's work. If, however, the learned professor redistributes his time, he can confine his operating to the rarities and the exceptional problems, in which only he and a few like him have experience, while a major portion of his time is devoted to training those general surgeons who are interested, to tackle safely and optimally the troublesome and unusual conditions which *will* crop up in their own districts from time to time. This training may be by means of courses and demonstration operations attended by only *very* small numbers of consultants for genuinely individual teaching, and also perhaps by means of the occasional visit to a DGH, to operate on a problem case together with the referring surgeon. The large teaching hospitals and major specialist units teach undergraduates and trainee specialists; one function of the highly specialized centre of excellence should be the continuing education of interested consultant surgeons throughout the land, training them to treat a larger proportion of their own difficult but interesting cases satisfactorily, rather than simply removing the patients, often far from home, and treating them without teaching anyone except a handful of future super-specialists. The general surgical consultants will require study leave to attend such courses, and this plus occasional visits by the super-specialist to 'share' a case should be tremendously stimulating for the hard-working, practical consultant. And what a reassurance to the patient to know that anything except the rarest of conditions can be quite adequately treated within his own district or region, and that, should he be unfortunate enough to suffer from a rarity, communications and relations between his local hospital and the specialist centre will be good, and the super-specialist, no longer over-burdened with more routine problems, will have time available to treat him.

Will the super-specialist then be a different sort of man from the general surgeon? Different, yes, but *not* superior. The more highly specialized the practitioner becomes, the more must he forget the boundaries between disciplines and the more his practice of medicine must become a science, so that his narrower field, by virtue of its greater depth, contains the same volume of knowledge and wisdom. The paediatric cardiac surgeon will have a knowledge of medical cardiology matching that of any physician; his medical counterpart, without actually operating, will be familiar with every detail of operative possibilities. Both will make extensive use of scientific methods in investigating patients, in monitoring their progress throughout treatment, and in applying clinical knowledge to research projects and vice versa; and of course these two men maintain close contacts with each other and with other specialist colleagues, for example in related areas of radiology and anaesthetics. Much of this super-specialist's time will be spent in consultative and investigative work, while his operating, although highly skilled and demanding of all his concentration, is limited in scope. The general surgeon, while he also must be to some extent a physician, and will use scientific methods in investigating many patients, spends a large part of his time in dealing with, and making decisions upon, relatively straightforward practical problems, and in operating skilfully on these with highly satisfactory results for the patient. While he may, to put it bluntly, have less time to think and to ponder, he is dealing in the main with people whose need is not for an intellectual, but for a man of rapid, sound decision based on knowledge and wisdom, and of skill in a far more varied range of surgical technique, which by that very variety provides satisfaction for the executor. If these two men are both to work usefully within our Health Service, there is no place for their labelling each other 'unthinking carpenter' and 'inefficient boffin' and the like; they must recognize the need for, and the worth of, their separate roles, and complement each other for the benefit of the patient: the specialist teaching the generalist so that the latter may then safely remove part of the former's practical load. Most general surgeons will then have a certain specialist interest to follow, and may use it to help colleagues with awkward cases, but all should retain their interest and practical skill in all routine surgical procedures. Discussions between surgeons with different interests should be deliberately fostered, to ensure that 'special interests' do not become isolated, and that important progress never goes unnoticed; it goes without saying, of course, that continued good communications within and without the NHS and the United Kingdom are vital.

Just as it is at last being recognized that general practice is a peculiarly 'special' specialty with its own peculiar demands, so must the future general surgeon be seen as specializing in the sort of activity described, of wide-ranging diagnosis, selection, and decision, and varied technical skills.

The major specialist surgical fields should remain in a separate category: those fields in which the range of techniques and instruments is sufficiently 'special', and yet the number of patients sufficiently large, to justify a unit for this purpose, at least in each region, and indeed in many district general hospitals, as with orthopaedic surgery. Thus the patient need never travel far for the help he needs. The men practising these major specialties are in a category similar to that of the general surgeon, in that patients are referred to them direct, but with surgical pathology of a particular type or in a particular anatomical area; the range of techniques may be rather less wide but is still varied. Here again there is no superiority or inferiority, but difference.

There remains what must now be the smallest category, although the field of work covered is the largest: this is the surgeon who is prepared to tackle any problem in the whole range of surgical practice. He will operate as necessary upon ears, heads, chests, bones, uteri, skin lesions, even eyes; he accepts that his results will never *quite* match those of each specialist but continues striving to make them do so. Regular consultations with colleagues play little or no part in his life, as the fact of his being obliged to cover such a range implies that he is working in comparative isolation. He therefore has more time for reading, and is dependent, in his endeavours, on good books and up-to-date journals.

Is there any place in the NHS for such a man? Should *any* of the population of our country be dependent on this less-than-optimum standard? Ideally, of course, no: but there are still, and by the nature of our geography will continue to be, places where communications are such that the safest policy is to have such a man on the spot, and where, even in the non-emergency situation or when transport facilities have improved, many patients will be happy to accept the standard offered locally as the condition for remaining on familiar territory. Thus it seems that in the foreseeable future this need will remain in such places as the Outer Hebrides, Orkney, and Shetland. Perhaps the greatest reassurance for these populations is that almost invariably the men who undertake such responsibilities are very conscious of them, and spare no effort to ensure that their patients do not suffer because of the surgeon's lack of specialization. The NHS already pursues for them an enlightened policy of study leave, refresher courses, and locum provisions; this policy must of course be maintained. (The work of doctors accompanying expeditions or ocean-going vessels may be comparable, but is usually for a limited period and covers only emergency situations.)

The other environment in which this most 'general' of surgeons may work (usually with even greater dedication and less help) is in remote parts of developing countries overseas. Is overseas work in any way relevant to the British Health Service of the future? What categories of surgeon engage in it? In the main, only two: from opposite ends of the spectrum. The super-specialist goes out from his centre of excellence to help train aspiring super-specialists in countries whose medical development is progressing rapidly towards the standards found in Britain. This is a temporary visit, not usually directed at benefiting our Health Service, except by the prestige gained by demonstrations of the standard of training which it provides. But the very general surgeon, usually a permanent or long-term worker, has also been trained by our Health Service, and it is doubtful if any other Service could provide him, should he deliberately seek it, with such a broad training as can ours. Like our other NHS emissary, this man must have his own brand of excellence. Yet, having gone, he is largely forgotten by his erstwhile colleagues who practise their several specialties within the comfort and security of the NHS; or he is dubbed a 'dilettante', or worse, a 'parasite' who has abdicated his responsibility to the country which trained him. Not so: this man is struggling to introduce United Kingdom

Health Service standards among people who would otherwise be denied anything even remotely approaching them. He is likely to make greater conscious efforts to keep up to date than do many of his UK colleagues. In his conscience, he has a wider-than-national responsibility; he had the good fortune to be born into a nation which was able to train him, and he sees his duty as being towards his fellow men of less fortunate birth, for at least a part of his working life. Despite his background and his standards, he will be fighting against odds never imagined by home-based colleagues: non-availability of drugs and equipment, ignorance and superstitious non-co-operation among patients; and in those with an early sophistication, just as many neuroses and trivia as he would see in UK, plus the problem of distinguishing between genuine poor and those who will try to use him as a 'soft touch' . . . Of course he will feel twinges of envy for those who have all facilities at hand, and basic security despite the rigours of the careers race. Perhaps I should allow one of these to express the philosophy: this sonnet, headed 'A Mission Surgeon's Thoughts, on his Diary', by an anonymous British surgeon working in a remote part of Asia, was found in another, less remote mission:

One hundred operated in five weeks,
Running the gamut of each Surgeon's sphere,
One thousand wait—can *I* give what each seeks?
Can England's standards hope to prosper here?

My native land—for this then was I trained?
I serve a race who do not know its worth;
Nothing the land which nurtured me has gained
Since for the world's far corners I set forth.

And yet, although no gold, something I earn
For that bright land which scarcely saw me go:
Untutored thousands here from me *may* learn
That caring which my race would have them know.

Joy within duty—nothing more I ask,
For God and for my fellow men the task.

Perhaps this man ought to return eventually to work within the NHS; if he does, will it be able to recognize his special gifts and experience . . . to use his unique contribution?

For surgical training in the future there must necessarily be a parallel pattern, geared to each and all of these categories.

We may first exclude from any formal scheme the fifth of our surgical prototypes, who will almost certainly wish to 'manage' his own training scheme, learning as much as possible of many specialties in the time available to him. It is to be hoped that NHS training at the most junior levels will never be so rigid that he cannot do this other than in a supernumerary capacity, which would be a pitiful waste of his energies and his professional devotion. Having worked in a number of different junior posts, he will leave the environment of most of his colleagues, possibly reappearing at intervals for professional refreshment.

The other four surgeons will set forth on postgraduate training which is almost identical in its early stages: after graduation they must all learn to become clinical doctors, and are likely to include in this clinical apprenticeship a high percentage of surgical work, and to devote much study time to pursuit of surgical interests and study of surgical writings. Thereafter, however, the present system could with advantage be altered. *All* surgeons today are trained to a fairly high level and for a considerable time in general surgery, and only later do the specialists *begin* to specialize. It seems doubtful whether this is necessary for the major surgical specialties. Does the budding orthopaedic, plastic, or neurological surgeon really benefit by spending a number of years in work which is principally in the abdomen? Is present-day 'general surgery' a necessary basis for orthopaedic surgery, any more than orthopaedic surgery is essential to the training of the general surgeon? Slightly more, perhaps, but only slightly. The time at present spent in general surgery is surely unnecessarily long, frustrating for the intending specialist once his intentions are definite, and an inefficient use of the NHS's time. Not only this, the fact that the specialist must *thereafter* learn his specialty, his total training being therefore longer than that of his general surgical colleague (as is the present plan for higher surgical training), encourages him in a sense of superiority to the general surgeon in intellect and skill. In reality, of course, neither should ever consider himself completely trained; both will surely accept that they continue to learn in their respective fields throughout their practising lives. The specialist surgeon, however, while doing this, is unlikely to keep fully abreast of knowledge or to continue practice in general surgery, and cannot for long justify a claim to know as much as his general surgeon colleague, plus some more. If his early years are thus largely wasted, would it not be better to allow him to limit his interest rather earlier in training to his chosen field, if it is one of these major branches which are unlikely ever to return within the scope of general surgery? (Basic surgical principles, introduced in general surgery, may be further taught in any major surgical field.) This would further confirm general surgery as a *different* specialty rather than a less highly skilled one, again comparable to the specialty of general practice in the wider field of medicine.

Here I may perhaps be forgiven for a brief digression from my topic of surgery in the future of the NHS. The preceding paragraph assumes a majority of graduates who have already made a definite choice, not only of major discipline but of major subspecialty, before or at an early stage in postgraduate training. This may appear inconsistent with the eminently sensible current trend away from trying to cram 'a bit of everything' into the undergraduate medical curriculum (a policy no longer feasible in the ever-widening range of medical knowledge if the new graduate is to have a useful depth of knowledge of anything). But if many subspecialties are excluded from the undergraduate curriculum, whence will their new recruits come? There is little doubt that the first career choice of most graduates is from the specialties to which they have been exposed before graduation. In the past this realization has led many 'specialist' teachers to condense far too much information into a limited ration of undergraduate time, thus confusing and in fact deterring the student. If, however, the student has a sound education in the basic concepts and major disciplines of medicine, and preferably also some training in the ethics and philosophy of his profession, he does not require a vast wealth of detail to attract his attention to a particular specialty. He must, of course, hear of its existence, why it exists, and broadly what it encompasses, but once his attention is caught he will himself seek out further detail until *he* decides he has sufficient information to pursue or reject a specialist field. The problem therefore is one of demonstrating to the student at a receptive and reasonably informed stage the various choices open to him after graduation. Experiments have been in progress for some years with 'Careers Fairs': many on a national basis. The idea is an attractive one, but potentially more than attractive. It should not be too difficult (assuming increasing university/hospital liaison in future) for *every* university or medical school to mount an annual Careers Fair. It need not be elaborate or costly, and the various specialists, both clinical and non-clinical, would undoubtedly enjoy preparing a display of their own chosen spheres of action in such a way as to attract recruits. If attendance at this 'Fair' replaced all other teaching, for perhaps a day or two, for students near the beginning of their clinical course, and again during the final year, at a time when they were not under pressure from imminent examinations, many would take a more intelligent and intense interest in certain fields during those clinical years, and a majority would have made an educated choice by the time of graduation, thus avoiding wastage of their own time and the Service's by subsequent indecision. 'Elective' periods in final year, available in specialties not otherwise taught to undergraduates, could further foster such decisions. The resultant increased efficiency of postgraduate training might enable its length to be safely reduced, without lowering standards.

Returning now to the postgraduate trainee surgeon, we consider our two remaining groups.

The super-specialist must perforce be trained initially as a general surgeon, if only because his super-specialty does not exist alone in most centres where postgraduates are trained. Only a few openings will be available for full-time aspirants to the exclusive field, at the centre of excellence; which is appropriate since only a few such super-specialists are required by the NHS. The total training will therefore tend to be longer than that of other surgeons, the man being fully or almost fully trained before confining himself to his specialty. Such prolongation should be acceptable to one whose future will be concerned mainly with rarities; one must allow time to see any significant number of cases of rare conditions. While he is less busy clinically in his later training years, he will doubtless be involved in research work (of which subject more later). But while pursuing knowledge in depth, he will not retain the breadth of knowledge and skill of those whom he may feel he 'left behind' in general surgery; he has no reason for any feeling of superiority, and as already suggested must endeavour to share his specialized skills as far as is practicable, for the benefit of the community and of his colleagues.

The general surgeon with a special interest must, of course, have completed a general surgical training. He may have developed and nurtured his special interest during that training; if fortunate he may have been able, during or after training, to work full-time for a limited period in a super-specialist unit of his choice. He may even have embarked on super-specialist training, only to find that it did not provide sufficient variety to satisfy him. On the other hand, his interest in one system may develop gradually, during his working-consultant life. Whatever the scheme he employs, this man's special interest must remain an *option*; he must be placed under no obligation or compulsion to sit examinations or undergo assessments in it unless he so chooses: he has already been fully assessed as a general surgeon and may remain simply that if he so wishes. Such possibilities for maintaining some special interest should, however, be stimulating for him, especially if he is further taught and encouraged at intervals, and treated as an equal, by the super-specialist.

What of research? As now, the super-specialists in the centres of excellence will be the spearhead of medical progress, inasmuch as most progress now is highly scientific and detailed in technique, and work towards it time-consuming. But the general surgeon still can and should help to expand the wider bounds of medical knowledge by clinical studies and clinical research. Many will do this; and while some will find or make time for some scientific research also, none should feel obliged to embark upon such work, wasting the Service's valuable time and money in some contrived scientific project because those responsible for career advancement apparently expect it. The Service *must* fight this tendency if it recognizes the general surgeon as a different but not inferior being, who will have had ample undergraduate training in scientific method to equip him as a clinical surgeon. Those who do require such training (the super-specialist and the non-clinical specialist) will have research methods included in their specialized training.

One further point: relationships with private practice. Whatever one feels about the continuing *need* for this, it seems probable there will always be a *demand*, and a nation which believes in personal liberty seems likely to continue at least to permit it. But as a profession whose basis is humanitarian, we must guard against ever equating centres of excellence with centres of private practice. The only justification for super-specialism in a country which has a National Health Service lies in its being available whenever, and in whomsoever, the need or the rare condition arises; it surely cannot, in our profession or in our society, be ethically acceptable if it becomes 'extra skill for extra money'.

Such, then, is a possible pattern for the future of surgery in the NHS; and it is the more likely to succeed in that it is akin to what has already evolved in response to the needs of the community. In the lead is the super-specialist, continually training able general surgeons and major-specialist surgeons who are interested in his field, often using their own problem cases as training material, so that they may extend the areas in which they can cope, leaving him relatively free to concentrate on the rarest problems and to push forward the frontiers of knowledge by his research; in the centre, those same general surgeons, with their major-specialist colleagues alongside, coping efficiently with the vast range of routine surgery, and increasingly, as led by the super-specialists, extending that range, possibly developing a special interest, possibly active in clinical research; at the margins of the Health Service and beyond, the pioneer-clinician for whom 'general' means all-comprehensive. There is no tail to our distribution, as none can be deemed to lag behind or be in any way inferior.

One might ask whether it is realistic to plan a rational pattern for the future of surgery, when the pattern of pathology may at any time undergo a dramatic change, such as the oft-cited possible discovery of a cure for malignant disease, or perhaps the finding of some means of dissolving various calculi. Such possibilities are by no means new; throughout the history of medicine old diseases have been conquered, and by this 'unmasking', or by extending knowledge, or by new environmental influences, new ones have appeared to replace them and pose fresh problems. Even present patterns are in a state of transition: witness the emerging specialty of traumatology, whose pathology has become too varied for continued inclusion within orthopaedics, and whose practitioners need a knowledge of emergency diagnosis and primary treatment for every surgical specialty but must then be prepared to decide the priority order of subsequent treatment and call appropriate colleagues. Witness transplant surgery, in which those who might until recently have been surgical urologists or hepatologists have had to join forces, learning each other's language anew where there was no previous overlap. Witness also the removal of vast amounts of thoracic surgery for tuberculosis and other infection, and its replacement by even more vast amounts for bronchial carcinoma; if this last were overcome, thoracic surgery (other than cardiac) *might* shrink to a level at which it could be returned within the ambit of general surgery, possibly as a 'special interest'. Thus the single specialty and subspecialty boundaries may and indeed must keep changing as pathological emphases alter, and some fields may become medical disciplines rather than surgical; research, too, may turn to less dramatic but nevertheless desperately cruel diseases, if and when 'killer' diseases are overcome and if they are not replaced by others equally lethal. But our over-all scheme for the entire discipline of surgery may withstand such fluctuations and still provide a comprehensive and logical service.

It has been suggested—hard to imagine with the advance of transplant surgery—that all surgery will one day be completely obsolete. Yet the advance of knowledge and of techniques, and the changing environment, have to our day kept the potential for cure constantly ahead of the rate of vanishing disease: thus far we continue to be necessary. Any state, however happy for humanity, in which it is in no circumstance necessary to pick up a knife or a needle and thread to alleviate some human ill, is so remote as to be impossible to envisage; and as long as such methods of treatment are needed, so long will men come forward who, finding satisfaction in using hand as well as mind in the service of their suffering fellows, will be proud of the designation 'surgeon'.

The next decade in general practice

ERIC GAMBRILL

ERIC GAMBRILL
MB, BS, MRCGP
General practitioner

The next decade in general practice

Ten years ago I had just entered general practice as a raw trainee, fresh from my student days and a succession of busy and stimulating junior hospital posts. I had never before visited a general practice either as a medical student or as a doctor.

My trainer was a kindly man in his early 60s, who worked from a surgery attached to his own home with one part-time partner. There was no appointment system, no special clinics, no practice nurse, no receptionist in the evenings, no typewriter, no dictaphone, no special equipment, and no age-sex or disease register. In my whole year I did not see or communicate with a health visitor, let alone a social worker. On occasion I did meet the district nurse by chance in a patient's home. The surgery was clean and nicely decorated, the waiting-room was warm and cosy and all the running costs came, in effect, directly out of my trainer's pocket.

He was clinically very astute and taught me much about the different skills and emphases required to practise clinical medicine in primary care. His knowledge and experience of psychological problems was immense and since my medical education had been almost totally deficient in this respect the learning situation was immensely valuable. It was he who introduced me to Michael Balint's classic book, *The Doctor, his Patient and the Illness*. He also taught me that to be a good doctor one should never cease to be a good student and together we attended many sessions at which hospital specialists lectured GPs about rare, unusual, and 'interesting' diseases.

The patients came to us with the usual variety of problems and symptoms with which any family doctor is familiar. The contraceptive pill had only come into general use quite recently and it was still considered something of a gamble by most women and viewed with grave suspicion by many doctors. Requests for abortion were almost unknown and those that did occur were arranged without our knowledge. We attended home deliveries and fervently hoped we should never need the flying-squad. Facilities for performing and reporting on cervical smears had just been made available by the local hospital. We had the early thiazides but no frusemide, no beta-blockers, no sodium cromoglycate, and the latest hypotensive in general use was guanethidine. The barbiturates were still by far the most common sedatives and tranquillizers in use and antidepressives were in their infancy.

In the academic field there was one Professor of General Practice in the whole of the UK and just a handful of places on vocational training schemes. The College of General Practitioners had been developing for twelve years and the report of the committee chaired by a past-president, Dr (now Dame) Annis Gillie had reported on *The Field of Work of the Family Doctor*. The over-all morale of general practice was low and the level of remuneration inadequate, but the signs of constructive change which were to develop into the Family Doctor's Charter were already apparent.

My purpose in describing in some detail a first-class practice of the traditional type as it existed ten years ago, and as some still exist today, is to draw attention to those excellent features which must not be lost sight of in the future development of general practice. Changes are occurring gradually in the morbidity and mortality patterns of disease, in the types of problems which patients consider suitable to present to their doctors, in the training and further professional development of the new generation of family doctors, in the organization of primary medical care, in our relationships with other workers in the health and social welfare fields, in our relationships with specialists and other vital members of the hospital team, and in our whole approach to research and academic development in our specialty. We should consider in some detail how these developments may be integrated into the general provision of high-quality primary medical care in the UK, with some attempt to compare and contrast these with parallel developments in other countries and other systems of medical care.

As we look towards the next decade we must first consider whether there are likely to be any major shifts in the nature and severity of illness presented to the GP. In the Royal College of General Practitioners' publication, *Present State and Future Needs of General Practice* (8), an attempt has been made to compile from a variety of sources a composite picture of the conditions which a hypothetical average GP with an average list of 2,500 patients may expect to see in the course of one year. Figures derived from urban and suburban practices in North America and Australasia suggest that the pattern is similar in these communities.

TABLE 1

Persons consulting for minor illnesses in a year in a hypothetical average practice of 2,500

Conditions	*Consultations per 2,500 patients*
General	
Upper respiratory infections	500
Emotional disorders	300
Gastro-intestinal disorders	250
Skin disorders	225
Specific	
Acute tonsillitis	100
Acute otitis media	75
Cerumen	50
Acute urinary infections	50
'Acute back' syndrome	50
Migraine	30
Hay fever	25

Source: Present State and Future Needs of General Practice (third edition, 1973).

As may be seen from Tables 1–6 the largest single group of conditions are those which are classified as minor or self-limiting, with no risk to life or permanent disability. That is not to dismiss them as 'trivia' since they may well occasion the patient or parent considerable discomfort, inconvenience, and anxiety, in addition to requiring a considerable degree of diagnostic sophistication in order to separate out the early signs of serious illness which are often almost indistinguishable from those of minor illness (1, 2, 3).

It seems most unlikely that any of these common conditions will diminish in frequency over the next decade. Indeed, it may well be that new technological developments may occur which will increase public demand. If a really effective antiviral agent became available enormous pressure would be placed on our primary care services, since it is known that at present less than one in four symptoms experienced by members of the general population are brought to the doctor. This is probably in the correct belief that there is at present little that we can do for them that they cannot do for themselves (45). Self-medication at the present time accounts for one-third of the national drug bill of £300 million in any one year. There is some evidence, however, that much self-medication is uninformed and inappropriate, and a research study is at present under way which is intended to investigate patterns of self-care. There may be scope here for education at school and directly by the doctor or nurse in the management of minor illness which would reduce the workload to some extent.

Turning to the table of acute major illnesses (Table 2), it is

TABLE 2

Persons consulting for acute major (life threatening) illnesses in a hypothetical average practice of 2,500.

Condition		*Consultations per 2,500 patients*
Acute bronchitis and pneumonia		50
Severe depression		12
Acute myocardial infarction		7
Acute appendicitis		5
Acute strokes		5
All new cancers		5
Cancer of lung	1–2 per year	
Cancer of breast	1 per year	
Cancer of large bowel	2 every 3 years	
Cancer of stomach	1 every 2 years	
Cancer of bladder	1 every 3 years	
Cancer of cervix	1 every 3 years	
Cancer of ovary	1 every 5 years	
Cancer of oesophagus	1 every 7 years	
Cancer of brain	1 every 10 years	
Cancer of uterine body	1 every 12 years	
Lymphadenoma	1 every 15 years	
Cancer of thyroid	1 every 20 years	
Suicidal attempts		3
Deaths in road traffic accidents		1 every 3 years
Suicide		1 every 4 years

Source: Present State and Future Needs of General Practice (third edition, 1973).

again difficult to see any profound changes in their pattern and incidence. Prompt and effective antibiotic therapy has already reduced the mortality from acute pulmonary infections almost to zero except in the elderly and in those already chronically ill with chest or cardiovascular disease. Severe depression presents a problem in case-finding especially among the elderly, and this is important because it is so eminently treatable. The epidemic of cardiovascular disease which is at present rife in the affluent societies of the world seems unlikely to abate within the next decade although in the longer term a change in our eating and smoking habits may help. The over-all incidence of malignant disease seems likely to increase, although the relative frequency of cancer occurring in different organs will continue to depend on multiple epidemiological variables.

What of those patients suffering from chronic illnesses and those with social handicaps (Tables 3 and 4)? Many of them fall

TABLE 3

Persons consulting for chronic illness in a year in a hypothetical average practice of 2,500

Conditions		*Consultations per 2,500 patients*
Chronic rheumatism		100
Chronic rheumatoid arthritis	10	
Chronic osteo-arthrosis of hips	5	
Chronic mental illness		55
Chronic bronchitis		50
Anaemia: iron deficiency		40
Anaemia: pernicious anaemia		3
Chronic heart failure		30
High blood pressure		25
Asthma		25
Peptic ulcer		25
Coronary artery disease		20
Cerebrovascular disease		15
Epilepsy		10
Diabetes		10
Parkinsonism		3
Multiple sclerosis		2
Chronic pyelonephritis		Less than 1
Tuberculosis		Less than 1

Source: Present State and Future Needs of General Practice (third edition, 1973).

TABLE 4

Social pathology in a population of 2,500

Conditions	*Persons*
Aged over 65	350
Poverty: receiving Supplementary Social Security Benefits	150
Aged over 75	100
Severe physical handicaps	70
Broken homes: one parent families with children under 15	60
Male homosexuals (estimated according to West, 1968)	50
Chronic alcoholics (Edwards, 1968)	5 (known) 25 (unknown)
Deaf (requiring hearing aids)	25
Severe mental handicaps	10
Blind (registered)	7
Problem families	5–10
Juvenile delinquents	5–7
Divorce	3–4
Illegitimate births	3
Adults in prison	1

Source: Present State and Future Needs of General Practice (third edition, 1973).

into both groups; the chronically ill are often poor and the poor are more likely to be chronically ill. Here is the field, above all, in which the need for teamwork at the level of primary care, both medical and social, has become increasingly apparent. Is there any real hope that the next decade will see a lessening of this tremendous burden on these unfortunate people? Doubtless the technical management of the rheumatic diseases will improve; new drugs, new surgical techniques and improved rehabilitation services will go some way to help but it seems premature to hope for a radical new approach to prevention and treatment. Cleaner air and a change in smoking habits may diminish chronic respiratory problems, and the management of cardiac failure, hypertension, epilepsy, and diabetes mellitus could be and should be improved. There may be a place for selective presymptomatic screening for a limited range of chronic diseases. New drugs, and, even more important, the correct use and control of established

TABLE 5

Congenital disorders (Carter, 1969) expected in a population of 2,500

Condition	*Expected in a population of 2,500*	
Congenital heart lesion	1 new patient every	5 years
Pyloric stenosis	1 new patient every	7 years
Talipes	1 new patient every	7 years
Spina bifida	1 new patient every	7 years
Mongolism	1 new patient every	10 years
Anencephaly	1 new patient every	10 years
Cleft palate	1 new patient every	20 years
Dislocation of hip	1 new patient every	20 years
Phenylketonuria	1 new patient every	200 years

Source: Present State and Future Needs of General Practice (third edition, 1973).

TABLE 6

Vital statistics in a population of 2,500

Annual vital statistics in a population of 2,500		*Numbers*
Marriages		17
Divorces		3–4
Pregnancies		40
Primipara	15	
Termination of pregnancy (NHS: 3), (Private: 3)	6	
Delivered at home	4	
Illegitimate	3	
Forceps deliveries	3	
Caesarean section	1–2	
Stillbirth	1	
Deaths		26
Cardiovascular	10	
Cancer	5	
Strokes	4	
Accidents	1	
Children under 15		600
Aged over 65		350

Source: Digest of Health Statistics 1971 (HMSO).

drugs will help, but the over-all incidence seems unlikely to decline.

With our ageing population the number of elderly people handicapped by strokes, rheumatic disease, and other chronic degenerative diseases will rise and this will throw a tremendous burden on their families, the community health and social workers, and all forms of hospital and residential accommodation. The tendency towards more active treatment and community care of the chronic mentally ill will inevitably involve the GP more deeply in the long-term management of these conditions.

What are the implications for the GP in these trends of morbidity and mortality? How should they affect his role and training? What are his needs in terms of colleagues, staff, tools, organization, and support? Finally, how shall we evaluate our work and effort and learn whether we are using our limited resources to maximum effect?

In 1969, a working party set up by the Royal College of General Practitioners to study and report on the educational needs of the future GP proposed a job definition which has become widely accepted. It does not differ in essentials from job definitions proposed by other academic bodies of family medicine around the world.

JOB DEFINITION

The general practitioner is a doctor who provides personal, primary and continuing medical care to individuals and families. He may attend his patients in their homes, in his consulting-room or sometimes in hospital. He accepts the responsibility for making an initial decision on every problem his patient may present to him, consulting with specialists when he thinks it appropriate to do so. He will usually work in a group with other general practitioners, from premises that are built or modified for the purpose, with the help of paramedical colleagues, adequate secretarial staff, and all the equipment which is necessary. Even if he is in single-handed practice, he will work in a team and delegate when necessary. His diagnosis will be composed in physical, psychological and social terms. He will intervene educationally, preventively and therapeutically to promote his patient's health.

This job definition tells us a great deal about the expected place, role, and function of the general practitioner in Britain during the next decade and beyond.

Let us examine it in more detail.

'The general practitioner is a doctor . . .'

This statement may seem self-evident but it has been seriously suggested that the level of care which lies between self-medication and specialist diagnosis and treatment requires no more than a specially trained nurse or medical assistant. In poor and developing nations, where the bulk of primary health care is concerned with the prevention and treatment of widespread infectious diseases, with malnutrition, and with the implementation of public health policy, and where national resources are severely limited this is the only efficient way to provide primary care. The 'barefoot doctors' of China and the medical assistant in Zambia are good examples of this type of worker.

In the more affluent countries, both east and west, the health problems at primary care level are utterly different, as has been demonstrated earlier, and the need is for a doctor who has shared his basic medical training with his peers in the specialist fields and then undergone a course of postgraduate training to equip him with the requisite knowledge, skills, and attitudes to function effectively in his chosen discipline. This is not to deny that the scope for delegation to, and co-operation with, other health workers is considerable and the team concept will be explored in detail later.

'. . . who provides personal, primary and continuing medical care to individuals and families.'

This implies a dimension of knowledge of, concern for, and responsibility to the patient which is an integral part of the best of traditional British general practice. It is sadly lacking in those systems of primary medical care which are based on the emergency rooms and multi-specialist clinics of large hospitals.

Most of the urban poor of the USA are cared for in this way and even their more affluent brethren often have no single doctor whom they know personally and to whom they can turn for any medical advice. Critics of group practice in the UK have been quick to suggest that this element of personal concern may be lacking but what evidence we have on the subject does not support this view (4). Nevertheless, it is a danger which must be resisted.

Direct access is the essential feature of primary or front-line care and the doctor–patient relationship is deepened and broadened by the fact that the same doctor is providing long-term and continuing care, often extending over many years, enabling him to evaluate symptoms and physical changes over long periods of time. The tradition of the GP having a defined list of patients for which he is continuously responsible is an important administrative result of this concept. I have had experience of working in other systems where responsibility is episodic and where some patients change doctors frequently, even during the course of the same illness. The results are unsatisfactory for patient and doctor alike and I would hope that there will be no moves in this direction in the UK.

The advantages of caring for an individual within his or her family setting, and of having first-hand knowledge of the marital, familial work, and neighbourhood environment in which he lives are obvious. Much of the ill-health dealt with by GPs stems from the failure of individuals to make appropriate adjustments to their life situations (6).

This may be the appropriate place to ventilate the old controversy of the generalist versus the specialoid: that is, the primary care doctor who limits his field of work to one age-group or specialty. Professor McKeown, who is a leading exponent of the specialoid approach believes that few generalists are now able to maintain a high level of expertise in all fields and that the individual family doctor should give way to the group care of families in which the paediatrician would look after the children, the physician would look after the adults, except for the adult females' obstetric care and gynaecological problems, and the geriatrician would look after the elderly. He suggests that this would enable the primary physician to participate in the secondary, hospital level of care to a much more significant extent and that the over-all quality of care would be enhanced. This type of career might prove attractive to some doctors who would otherwise emigrate or become disgruntled generalists.

It would be fair to say that this view is widely regarded as heretical by British GPs, except in a few outposts such as Guy's and Southampton, but there is no real evidence on which to base a considered judgement. Doubtless, experimentation will continue and there will certainly be an increasing tendency for some members of a group to develop special interests and expertise which will be made available to their partners. If the specialoid-group approach became established in the UK, it would be a significant improvement in the situation obtaining in the USA and USSR where the specialoids tend to work in isolation from each other, and where the dimensions of family care are often lost completely.

'He may attend his patients in their homes, in his consulting-room or sometimes in hospital.'

Indeed, he may attend his patients in their homes, but he is increasingly less likely to do so. Statistics and experience from a wide variety of practices in the UK, both urban and rural, have shown an almost universal decline in home-visiting, on average 60 per cent less than ten years ago (8). Major factors in this decline have been considered to be the wide availability of private transport, of private telephones, and of appointment systems. There has also been a good deal of propaganda from the profession and the DHSS in an attempt to persuade patients to attend surgery whenever possible. Experiments in the use of transport services in general practice have been sponsored by the DHSS but the costs per case seem relatively high (8). Since a home visit occupies on average three times as much expensive doctor-time as a surgery consultation, the economic advantages to the NHS are obvious. There is a danger, however, that excessive reduction in home-visiting would have deleterious effects on the condition of some patients and there is evidence from North America that it may also lead to an increased use of extremely expensive hospital beds for relatively trivial conditions.

The consulting-room has now become the focus of general practice since here may be found the staff, the records, the equipment, and the ancillary workers which help to provide the optimum conditions in which the doctor may work. The number of consultations per patient per year varies widely between two and seven, related to the geographical and social conditions of the practice and also to the personality and method of working which the doctor employs. It is interesting to note that average annual consultation rates in primary care vary from around five to six per year in North America and Australasia to between ten and twenty per year in Italy and Japan and it seems unlikely that there will be any marked change in consultation patterns in the UK over the next decade (8).

The relative brevity of the average consultation, six to seven minutes, is often a matter for criticism both by doctors and patients, but if time spent on routine check-ups is excluded, the average consultation time in primary care is of the same order all over the western world. There will never be as much time as we might wish for, although improving organization and the delegation of some routine work to ancillaries will help.

What of the relationship between the GP and the hospital? In what ways is it likely to change and develop over the next decade? What indeed are the functions of the modern district general hospital?

First, the hospital is the logical site for the centralization of diagnostic laboratories and radiological equipment. In this age of increasing sophistication and automation there is little place for the isolated unit. It is generally considered that a population of about 100,000 is required to use these facilities economically. Nevertheless, the fact that the facilities are geographically centred in the hospital does not mean that they should be regarded as the property of the hospital. Their function is to serve the whole medical community and open access for GPs is essential. The evidence is that GPs generally request straightforward and relatively cheap tests and X-rays and that the proportion of abnormal results is actually higher than in those investigations requested by the specialist units (8). The availability of an electrocardiography service has been shown to be of value but whenever possible the machine should be available within the primary care unit. The provision of an item-of-service payment, which could well be conditional on proven experience and education, would increase the informed use of the ECG in primary care.

Apart from these diagnostic services the district general hospital (DGH) also provides the physiotherapy and occupational therapy services which are required in the increasingly important field of rehabilitation. The correct use of these departments by GPs and their consultant colleagues is vital and projects such as geriatric day- and five-day hospitals depend heavily upon them.

Secondly, the hospital out-patient department is the traditional site for the location of the ambulatory specialist referral service, although it need not be the only one. The patient may be seen by the specialist in his home or in the practice centre. The referral rates to the various specialties vary widely among GPs and this is an aspect which requires further study.

What does the GP want when he refers a patient to an out-patient department? It may be that he is perplexed by a diagnostic problem and requests help. It may be that he has made the diagnosis and refers the patient for specialized treatment. This, of course, is particularly true in the surgical specialties which account for the largest proportion by far of out-patient referrals. It may be that the GP is confident of his diagnosis and treatment, but that the patient requests a second opinion, or it may be that the diagnosis is so serious that the GP feels the need for professional support and confirmation. Whatever the indication for referral it is incumbent on the GP to state clearly what he requires from the consultant and for the consultant to communicate relevant information and advice. Once the problem is solved or the treatment completed the patient should be referred back to his GP. Many hours are wasted by both doctors and patients when the patient is followed-up simultaneously by the GP and an ever-changing succession of junior hospital doctors. There is enormous scope for improvement in the arrangements for sharing of care between hospital clinic and GP along the lines pioneered by the obstetricians and GPs in the provision of shared antenatal and post-natal care. Diabetes mellitus, hypertension, rheumatoid arthritis, and post-gastrectomy surveillance are just a few examples which spring to mind. In Scotland a computerized scheme for follow-up of treated thyroid patients by GPs using a standard proforma and venepuncture kit has proved popular, efficient, and successful.

Surely the time has come when agreed criteria of good care in these chronic conditions can be standardized. The consultant clinic would then return to its proper role of initial assessment, stabilization and establishment of therapy, together with the management of problems which may arise in the course of treatment. There would need to be continuing opportunities for mutual education in these chronic conditions. A scheme for the care of diabetic patients in this way, with the establishment of mini-clinics within the group practices, was recently reported in the *British Medical Journal*. Investigation of the possibilities for shared care may well be an important task for the new health-care planning teams.

Thirdly, the DGH is the natural site for the postgraduate

centre, which should be the focus of the medical community in a district for educational, professional, and social contact.

Fourthly, there will be a continuing and probably increasing demand for GPs to work in the hospital as medical and clinical assistants in the specialist team. The GP can fulfil an important service need and at the same time develop a level of expertise in the specialty which will be of use to his partners and patients in the community. In order to be of maximum service value to the hospital he will be expected to practise for some years in a given specialty. From an educational point of view, however, there is much to be said for experimentation with shorter periods of attachment of GPs to relevant specialties, possibly on a rotational basis. Increasing numbers of hospitals for psychiatric and mentally subnormal patients are relying on GPs for the provision of general medical care to the patients, which is of benefit to both the hospital and the GP.

Fifthly, what should be the role of accident and emergency departments *vis-à-vis* the GP? Attendances at these departments almost doubled over the twenty years 1950–70. In what measure was this related to changes in the pattern of general practice? How are they to be staffed in view of the increasing shortage of junior medical staff prepared to apply for these jobs?

There is universal agreement that the primary function of an accident and emergency department must be to deal efficiently and quickly with major trauma and sudden major illness occurring at work or in the street. Patients, however, are increasingly referred by GPs for the treatment of minor trauma involving suturing and the setting of undisplaced fractures, especially in urban areas. This trend has been exacerbated since GPs have increasingly felt that the local department is better organized and equipped to deal with these problems and since these time-consuming jobs involve no extra payment. The same factors have resulted in increased referral rates for minor surgery such as opening abscesses, removing sebaceous cysts, and resecting toe-nails. With the advent of appointment systems in general practice, some of which have undoubtedly been too rigidly administered, a number of patients have become accustomed to drop in for instant diagnosis and treatment, whilst others have taken the opportunity of an unofficial second opinion. Still other patients are more inclined to go to accident and emergency departments at night and weekends than to disturb their own GP, in the mistaken belief that the departments are staffed on a shift-system with doctors waiting expectantly for work day and night. Some elements of the population in the centres of our large cities have always looked especially to the teaching hospitals to provide their primary care. They have not been dissuaded since this was often the only primary care experience available to the medical students. If we wish to change the present situation in the next decade it will require further data on the usage of accident and emergency departments, close co-operation between the responsible consultants and GPs in local areas and, most probably, changes in the remuneration system for GPs.

Sixthly, and most contentious of all, what will be the place of the GP in the DGH over the next decade. No-one would dispute the value of the GP's continuing contact with the patient while in hospital. The patient benefits from contact with his own personal medical adviser whom he knows and trusts and the specialist team benefit from the GP's knowledge of the previous medical history and the psychological and social background of the patient and his family. Here is an excellent opportunity for the mutual education of GPs, consultants, and junior hospital doctors. It would be helpful if all hospitals had a system which informed the GP when a patient is admitted from the waiting-list. Unfortunately, constraints of time and distance from the DGH will always make it difficult for some GPs to visit their patients regularly while in hospital, but all possible encouragement should be given.

At this point we must consider the nub of the problem. Should the GP have direct access to beds in the DGH in which to care for his own patients? Is there any evidence that the demand exists? In 1972, the Royal College of General Practitioners and the Royal College of Physicians published a joint report entitled, *The General Practitioner in the Hospital*, which suggested that there was a demand and a case to be made. It seems that, in general, younger doctors are more keen than older doctors to look after their patients in hospital and the lack of this facility has been postulated as one contributing cause of young doctors being unwilling to enter general practice in the UK. One reason for this may be the need to retain the umbilical cord to mother hospital, where they have been extensively, and often entirely, trained, but personal experience of vocationally trained young GPs at a recent conference in Edinburgh suggests that they, too, are in favour of further developments in this field.

What type of case might the GP wish to admit and care for himself? Reports suggest that the first criterion is that any patient whom he would normally care for at home, if adequate family and community support were available, should be admitted to a GP bed. These would be predominantly respiratory and cardiovascular conditions, particularly in elderly people. The second type of case is for terminal care, when the family is either unwilling or unable to continue care at home. It is often better to admit these patients locally where their family may visit them frequently than to send them miles away to even a first-class nursing home or terminal care unit. Another situation in which they might be used is in short-term care for the younger chronic sick in order to give the family a break or for a short period of intensive nursing care and physiotherapy. The evidence is that the average length of stay of patients in GP beds ranges from six to eighteen days, which is intermediate between that of the general medical and geriatric departments, as might be expected.

It is not envisaged that the GP would take direct responsibility for patients undergoing surgery or admitted to the intensive care unit as is sometimes the case in North America. Long-term trends, however, suggesting a diminution in the number of junior hospital doctors and an increase in the number of GPs, may produce a situation in which this type of involvement is encouraged. Paediatric and psychiatric admissions are generally considered to be unsuitable for GP care and long-stay geriatric and psychiatric patients should remain the responsibility of the relevant specialists.

So far we have been chiefly concerned with the place of the GP in the DGH. Is there a continuing need for cottage hospitals, community hospitals, or peripheral nursing units? The answer must be a qualified 'yes', at least in areas remote from a DGH, and Emrys Roberts and others have written cogently and passionately on the subject. In rural and suburban areas they will remain separate entities, although some have been developed with health centres on the same site. In urban areas GP beds should probably be situated within the DGH, although a concept of health centres with beds attached, staffed entirely by the community nursing service, has been proposed by Draper and his colleagues.

The involvement of the GP in hospital obstetrics is a special case. As home delivery has become more uncommon, now under 10 per cent of all births in the UK, the GP has tended to acquire hospital obstetric beds and 22 per cent of the obstetric beds in 1972 were for GP use, but 76 per cent of these were in units away from a DGH. Paradoxically, in this field where the GP has been most active in hospital, technical developments in the active management of labour and increasingly sophisticated forms of analgesia threaten his capability to remain in charge at the time of delivery. It may well be that the future pattern will be of shared antenatal and post-natal care between GP and obstetrician, with delivery in the specialist unit and an increasing tendency to early discharge of all healthy mothers and babies. It has always seemed to me ironic that we, who have one of the best community midwifery services in the world, keep our mothers and babies in hospital after normal delivery longer than almost any other nation. It may be that changes in the midwifery regulations and the organization of midwifery services are long overdue.

'He accepts the responsibility for making an initial decision on every problem his patient may present to him, consulting with specialists when he thinks it appropriate to do so.'

As a direct result of the family doctor offering personal, primary, and continuing medical care, and, in addition, often being the only professional person with whom many people are familiar, he is often approached by patients for advice on a range of topics outside of even the most liberal medical education. He will observe problems in the course of unravelling and exploring those 'illnesses' which have their roots in the non-physical sphere, which will require referral to, or contact with, other professionals and other agencies. These may include lawyers, social workers, probation officers, teachers, clergy, Samaritans, Citizens' Advice Bureaux, housing departments, social security departments, the disablement resettlement officers at the Department of Employment, employers, and industrial medical officers and a host of others. The future GP should be well versed in the range of skills and services which these agencies can provide, in addition to his knowledge of the special strengths and weaknesses of the medical specialists to whom he refers his patients.

'He will usually work in a group with other general practitioners, from premises that are built or modified for the purpose.'
The trend in the UK, though this is by no means universal in the western world, is toward group practice as may be seen from Table 7.

TABLE 7
Percentage of GPs working in various size groups in England and Wales (1948–71)

Year	*Single-handed*	*(No. of GPs)* 2	3	4	5	6+	*Total number of GPs*
1948	80						
1951	43	38	13	5	1	—	17,202
1954	38	35	16	7	3	1	18,552
1957	34	35	19	8	3	1	19,423
1960	31	34	21	9	3	2	19,914
1963	25	32	24	13	4	2	20,335
1966	30	24	24	15	5	2	19,832
1969	21	26	26	15	7	5	20,133
1971	23	27	17	8	8	5	20,600

Source: Annual Reports of the Department of Health and Social Security and Home and Health Department, Scotland.

The advantages to be gained from group practice are many and the potential of group practice for the over-all improvement of standards in primary medical care is considerable. One of the most widely criticized aspects of general practice as a professional and academic discipline is the professional isolation of the practitioner and the lack of any adequate system of quality control (10, 11).

While the hospital consultant is constantly under the critical eye of his junior staff and nurses and the junior hospital doctor is continually responsible to his chief, the GP, particularly the single-handed doctor, has virtually no external stimulus to the maintenance of high professional standards. This is not essential if the doctor concerned has the ability to monitor his own actions critically and be constantly aware of the dangers of stagnation and retrogression, but for most ordinary mortals critical and informative contact with colleagues is a vital part of professional development. This is particularly important in the setting of primary medical care in the UK where many practitioners have little or no direct contact with their hospital colleagues.

The development of postgraduate centres and official encouragement of continuing education has helped to some degree in encouraging contact, but formal meetings and courses are no substitute for the direct, day-to-day contact, discussion, co-operation, and education which should go on within the well-organized group practice. Some groups now engage in regular assessment of quality control within the practice, discussing the management of patients who have died, of newly diagnosed cases of serious disease and also holding discussions on notes selected at random by the staff. The aim is to see if the outcome of the condition could have been improved by earlier diagnosis or better management.

If such audits are conducted in an educational rather than a critical atmosphere they are extremely valuable methods of continuing education which are not available to the single-handed doctor. New ideas can be transmitted, new items of information shared and respect for the particular skills and emphasis of primary care medicine, rather than hospital-orientated medicine, engendered in the new entrants to general practice.

Even with the increasing numbers of new practitioners who have undergone an appropriate course of training for general practice there is much to be learnt during the first few years through constant contact with older and wiser doctors. They, in turn, benefit from exposure to young minds, critical and observant and able to contribute information on the newer techniques of hospital medicine. Such a valuable process is denied to the single-handed GP.

More refined and detailed methods of quality control such as those developed by Professor Spitzer at MacMaster University, Ontario, involving the use of tracer diseases and tracer drugs, together with the introduction of flow-charts and checklists to measure actual care as compared to ideal care will also be further developed and experimented with. The introduction of the problem-orientated medical record into general practice following the work of Metcalfe and others in developing the original methods of Weed, will allow for closer inspection of the process which is involved in high-quality primary medical care.

Other advantages of working in groups include benefit for the vocational training of young GPs, ease of attachment of para-medical staff, generally better organization, equipment, and secretarial help, and the ease of arranging rotas for holidays, nights, and weekends, thus reducing the need for reliance on deputizing services.

The Family Doctor Charter in 1966 provided a major impetus to the building of new group practice premises and the extensive alteration and improvement of old ones. This was achieved through the total reimbursement of rent and rates, with a notional agreed rent for privately owned premises, and through a system of guaranteed loans provided by the General Practice Finance Corporation, in addition to the provision of direct improvement grants by the DHSS.

The increase in the number of health centres provided by local authorities has been even more dramatic, rising from a total of 76 in the whole of England in 1968 to the present position where over 400 will soon be in operation and more than 10 per cent of all the GPs in the country will soon work from such a building. The biggest disappointment so far has been that most of the rehousing of primary medical care has been achieved in those areas, such as the counties and the county boroughs, which were already reasonably well served, whilst the central city areas in most need have been relatively neglected. The need is great for the development of health centres in these areas and the teaching-hospital could play a great part in developing primary care services in their own vicinity. The BMA Planning Unit Report No. 4 (6) made constructive suggestions regarding such developments.

'... *with the help of paramedical colleagues, adequate secretarial staff and all the equipment which is necessary.*'

One of the most important changes in general practice in the past decade has been the development of the team from an experimental attachment to the point where the health team is now 'a real, accepted and applied concept in community care' (8). Probably 50 per cent or more of health visitors, district nurses, and domiciliary midwives are now attached to GPs. It is to be hoped that the reorganization of the NHS will serve to accelerate and consolidate this tendency. We should be cautious, however, in assuming that administrative attachment alone will solve problems of communication and co-operation between these professionals. We should not be satisfied until they all work from the same premises, thoroughly understand the roles and functions of other members of the team and meet constantly to exchange ideas and information, discuss patients' problems, and co-operate fully in their joint tasks.

The attachment of health visitors has perhaps been the most outstanding success so far. With her unique background of nursing, midwifery, social, educational, and preventive skills and training she is ideally suited to work with the GP. No longer should she regard herself as responsible only for the preventive medical and social welfare of the preschool children. Every patient and every family in the practice is potentially her concern and responsibility. This may range through involvement in antenatal and post-natal clinics, care of the elderly, the chronic sick, problem families, and the multitude of part medical and part social and psychological problems which occur.

At present there is only one health visitor available to every three GPs, but I am convinced that the full potential of her contribution will not be realized until the ratio is one to one. It is to be hoped that future developments in nurse training in the wake of the Briggs' report will in no way jeopardize the future supply of these invaluable front-line workers.

By and large, the attachment of district nurses has not involved such profound changes in relationships since both doctors and nurses already had a fairly clear idea of each other's roles. The nurse, however, has tended to become much more involved in surgery work in addition to home nursing. Reedy has summarized the work which may be performed by both SRNs and SENs within the practice (8).

Opinions differ sharply on whether there is any place for a specially trained nurse to conduct initial consultations or home visits in selected cases, as has been described in the UK by Smith and Mottram (12). In the USA, nurse-practitioners and physicians' assistants capable of limited diagnosis and treatment under the over-all guidance of a doctor are being trained in small numbers, whilst in the USSR the *feldsher* has a long and honourable history. There are still doubts about the legal position of such workers but doubtless experimentation will continue. Practice nurses, employed and paid directly by the doctor, may be more suitable in this role, at least for the present.

The domiciliary midwife works better when attached to a

group of doctors, when she can share the antenatal and post-natal care at joint clinics. With the decline of home delivery this aspect of her work will diminish, but increasingly she is going into the hospital GP unit, conducting the delivery and returning mother and baby home early for continuing care. This system works well and is capable of considerable expansion and development.

A small number of social workers have been attached to groups of GPs and have reported on their experiences (13, 14).

It seems that her role is that of a specialist caseworker dealing with a relatively small number of complex and time-consuming problems. Unfortunately, the numbers of social workers are so limited and the demands on them so great that the best one can hope for in the next decade is for increased liaison between some social workers and group practices, perhaps with the social worker holding one or two sessions a week on the practice premises. Such an arrangement would give the two professions a chance to learn about each other's unique skills and divergent approach to problems, an educational process which is long overdue.

Social service departments now have responsibility for home helps, meals-on-wheels, and other vital social welfare services.

Direct reimbursement of 70 per cent of the salary of medical secretaries and receptionists has transformed the administrative side of general practice. Many group practices now employ a practice manager responsible for all the non-professional aspects of the practice, and efficient telephone, dictation and typing, reception, and appointment systems are commonplace. Age/sex and diagnostic registers capable of identifying groups of 'at-risk' patients are gradually spreading and there may well be a place in the future for area health authorities to provide teams of specially trained clerks to establish these in practices which require them. The training of secretarial staff is improving all the time and there will be increasing numbers of suitably trained girls emerging from the training colleges, having completed the courses organized by the Association of Medical Secretaries. In time a career-structure may develop spanning the various branches of the NHS but there will always be a need in general practice for mature, married women, employed part-time, on whom so many practices rely.

What type of equipment is required by the GP at his practice premises? Assuming open access to X-ray and pathology facilities there is no place for their location in primary medical care units. The electrocardiogram should become standard, with increased education in its interpretation and use available to GPs. Some simple test of pulmonary function, such as the Wright peak flow meter, is invaluable, and simple audiometric facilities could well become more widespread. No practice should be without a full range of dip and tablet urine tests, vaginal specula and proctoscopes, an accurate weighing machine for adults and babies, ear-syringing equipment, and a refrigerator. Considerable criticism has been levelled at the relative paucity of equipment available to the average British GP (10, 11), but the important factor is that the equipment should be used rationally and effectively, with full understanding of its limitation and value. When an item-of-service payment is made for diagnostic tests in some systems of medical care, the frequency of performance often bears little relation to the actual need for help in the clinical management of the patient.

'Even if he is in single-handed practice, he will work in a team and delegate when necessary.'

Not all groups of GPs are financial partners, although this is the normal pattern in the UK. The report of the committee chaired by Dr Harvard Davis on group practice stressed the importance of each doctor retaining his own list of patients who would normally see him whenever possible. It was further suggested that the long-term aim should be for a basic unit of primary medical care consisting of one doctor, one health visitor, one district nurse, and one secretary-receptionist.

Perhaps we shall ultimately return to a form of single-handed practice in which the team approach can be developed and organization and support services provided in the context of health-centre practice. Rural areas present special problems but even there all possible steps must be taken to avoid the professional isolation of the GP.

'His diagnoses will be composed in physical, psychological and social terms.'

It is essential that above all the GP should be a clinician competent to diagnose promptly acute and life-threatening illness and capable of managing the medical aspects of chronic illness (6). He must practise, however, against a background which presents him with many other problems and symptoms which cannot be understood in terms of disease and the processes of pathology in which he was trained as a student.

In the past, when there was little geographical mobility, social mobility, or indeed professional mobility, this knowledge of personality and social stress was acquired over long periods of time. In our increasingly mobile world patients and physicians are less likely to know each other for a lifetime and thus the need for an increase in the level of professional skills in interpersonal relationships, and in the application of knowledge gained from the behavioural sciences, particularly psychology and sociology, is a prerequisite for high-quality primary care. The Royal Commission on Medical Education made particular comment on 'the many witnesses who pointed to the increasing frustration and dissatisfaction of many GPs at their inability to deal with a substantial proportion of patients whose difficulties are psychological or social in origin'. The stress I have laid on the development of these newer skills is not intended to denigrate the importance of traditional clinical medicine, especially a thorough grounding in general medicine, geriatrics, paediatrics, and psychiatry which must be the bedrock of a primary physician's skill. It is not open, however, to the future GP to declare himself only prepared to deal with 'real medicine'. He is daily presented with undifferentiated problems which will not be solved by a firm declaration that nothing is physically wrong. The way in which the consultation is handled and the careful assessment of the patient's real problem may save both doctor and patient many hours, days, weeks, or months of anguish and the NHS considerable resources in needless investigation and therapy.

'He will intervene educationally, preventively and therapeutically to promote his patient's health.'

Once the correct diagnosis and assessment is made, the future management of the situation will become more rational. It may involve drug therapy, requiring the GP to be constantly up to date in the fast-changing field of therapeutics, it may involve educating the patient in regard to the nature of chronic disease and the limitations which the disease may put upon his or her life, it may require counselling and coming to terms with problems of personality and outlook which cannot be changed, or it may involve referral to a medical specialist or the mobilization of some of the wide range of social support services which are now available.

What of the GP's role in preventive medicine, in family planning, in screening for pre-symptomatic or unreported disease, and in the long-term follow-up of chronic illness? There is an increasing tendency for immunization and vaccination programmes for children to be based on health centres, with much of the routine work being performed by other members of the primary care team, and with organization and administrative support provided by the community physician as in the pioneering scheme in West Sussex described by Galloway. The tendency has been for practices to set aside special periods for immunization clinics and this has naturally led on to well-baby and infant welfare clinics being held jointly by the health visitor and the GP. This trend is logical, efficient, and must continue to develop. In some instances clinics for the developmental screening of infants and children, as described by Sheridan and others, have been established by enthusiasts, but it seems unlikely that they will become general unless a suitable item-of-service payment is made as a matter of public policy.

Such a payment is now under negotiation in regard to family planning services and it seems likely that interested and properly trained GPs will continue to expand the range and quality of contraceptive services provided. Integration of the present school health service with general practice is occurring in some areas and seems a logical development. Possible future developments in regard to shared obstetric care and the long-term follow-up of chronic disease have already been discussed. Hopefully the GP will increasingly think in terms of health education and disease prevention in his day-to-day work. The alteration of exercise, eating, drinking, smoking, drug, and reproductive habits would prevent or minimize more ill health than all the screening programmes will ever do. Who is in a better position than the GP to exercise such influence?

The pros and cons of screening for presymptomatic disease in general practice are a subject of continuing and increasing debate. In North America the regular health check-up, extending even to sigmoidoscopy and multiple biochemical tests, is an established part of the primary physician's work, but little effort has been made to evaluate the benefits of this approach. The potential cost in terms of professional time and resources is enormous, and great care must be taken to examine the evidence critically before embarking on any new screening procedure except on a carefully controlled experimental basis (15). The greatest success in the past was the use of mass miniature chest radiography in the detection of pulmonary tuberculosis but this is now a relatively rare condition in the general population. A good case can be made out for early detection of congenital dislocation of the hip, visual defects, deafness, and phenylketonuria in children, but the benefits of cervical cytology and screening for hypertension are less easy to evaluate. The screening of elderly patients for reversible disease is a popular new field at present, although the benefits may well be social and personal rather than strictly medical.

If there are further moves in the direction of anticipatory care it is important that lay and paramedical staff should be used as extensively as possible. Doctors are highly trained and expensive creatures, who soon tire of seeing healthy people in large numbers.

Having discussed at some length the future role and function of the GP and speculated about his place and relationship within the NHS, how are we to meet the educational challenge this presents?

First, what has general practice to contribute to undergraduate education? Professor Knox, at the Update International Symposium on Primary Medical Care, held in New York in 1973, listed the clinical aims as: (1) to widen the students' understanding of patterns of disease, (2) to demonstrate primary diagnosis and management, (3) to illustrate continuity of care, especially in chronic disease, (4) to demonstrate aspects of preventive medicine, and (5) to deepen the students' understanding of the doctor–patient relationship. He listed the professional aims as: (1) to allow the student to see family practice in action, (2) to afford the student the opportunity to consider possible changes in the pattern of medical care, and (3) to assist the medical school to promote an holistic approach to medicine.

Departments of general practice and family medicine are being established rapidly all over the western world. In the UK the

Scottish universities have led the way. This trend is likely to continue and accelerate since they have much to contribute to the education of all medical students. They also provide an appropriate forum for joint educational projects with other health and social workers in training. It is never too early to learn the nature and value of the skills of other professionals.

Some postgraduate experience in general practice would be invaluable for many specialists, especially perhaps community physicians, paediatricians, geriatricians, physicians, psychiatrists, and gynaecologists and it may be that in the future the equivalent of SHO posts in general practice will be established. This would go some way to recreate the understanding of the different range and perspectives of primary care which was lost when specialization from general practice ceased to be the norm.

The main educational effort, however, will inevitably be placed on the vocational training of young doctors for the specialty of primary medical care. An immense amount of study and research into educational methods and the development of a suitable syllabus has culminated in the publication of a book entitled *The Future General Practitioner—Learning and Teaching*, written by a working party of outstanding teachers appointed by the Royal College of General Practitioners. The detailed educational objectives have been arranged into five areas: (1) clinical practice: health and disease; (2) clinical practice: human development; (3) clinical practice: human behaviour; (4) medicine and society; (5) the practice.

There are at present over three hundred places a year available on vocational training schemes for general practice. The usual pattern is for the trainees to spend two years in relevant hospital posts and one year in the teaching practice, which may be in one block or divided into two periods of varying length. The schemes also involve regular seminars and discussion groups, and at least one year of a formal half-day or day-release course. Whilst these formal schemes will continue to grow and develop, there will also be some young doctors who prefer to follow their own schedules, preferably arranged in consultation with their regional postgraduate adviser in general practice, culminating in a final year in the teaching practice. Ultimately we shall require at least a thousand fully trained doctors a year to enter general practice.

The teaching practice is a new concept, ranging from the multi-function university teaching practice at one end of the spectrum to carefully chosen, predominantly service-oriented NHS practices at the other (16). The trainers and their practices are now selected by the regional postgraduate committees and the trainers are paid a substantial addition to their remuneration.

All the major medico-political groups have now accepted the principle of a minimum three-year training period for future GPs, and it is intended that this should be implemented by 1977 or as soon as possible after that date. Already there is a small vocational training allowance payable for the first ten years in independent practice and this goes some way to compensate for financial loss in the training years.

The examination for membership of the Royal College of General Practitioners is available as a voluntary test of competence in the discipline of general practice. Candidates must either have been fully registered for at least four years, of which not less than two years have been spent in general practice, or for at least three years if they have completed a vocational training scheme recognized by the college.

Continuing education for established GPs is also a rapidly developing field. The spread of purpose-built postgraduate centres and the appointment of GP advisers to clinical tutors should ensure that the educational material provided is relevant and varied. The Medical Recording Service of the RCGP has pioneered an extensive library of tape–slide teaching material and newer developments include videotape recordings and television transmissions. Specialty journals of general practice such as the *Journal of the Royal College of General Practitioners*, *The Practitioner*, and *Update*, are available in addition to the more general medical journals and increasing numbers of textbooks dealing with aspects of general practice are being written by GPs for GPs and other interested doctors. Ultimately only the GPs themselves can determine their own educational needs. There is as yet no suggestion of a formal re-accreditation system or re-examination at five-yearly intervals such as that adopted by the American Academy of Family Physicians.

The recent publication by the RCGP of *Oral Contraceptives and Health* has highlighted the immense potential for research in general practice. This first report is based on observations of

46,000 women, in 1,400 practices, over four years. It is doubtful if this study could have been carried out in such depth, or with such accuracy and continuity anywhere else in the world, but large co-operative studies are by no means the only way in which a GP may become involved in research. Interested GPs provide a mass of epidemiological data to national bodies and to research units including those of their own college. Individual epidemiological studies have yielded information of great value. Studies of many aspects of common and even relatively uncommon disease have been performed. The assessment and investigation of new drugs for use in general practice is carried out on a routine basis, and there is now a mass of published data on every conceivable organizational feature of general practice. The General Practitioner Research Club acts as a forum in the UK for all those who are interested. If general practice is to increase its prestige and status and contribute its rightful share of new medical knowledge there must be continuing research of quality performed.

General practitioners will also have an increasing part to play in the administration and advisory structure of the reorganized NHS. Individual GPs function at regional and area authority level and the GPs of each district elect their representatives on to the district medical committee, which in turn elects a GP to the district management team, together with a consultant. This is a new type of role for most GPs and one which requires suitable interest, aptitude, and training if it is to be successfully carried out. The GP members of the new, and potentially very important, health-care planning teams to be established in each district, will contribute in a direct way to the future integration of all aspects of health and social care, and hopefully these bodies will produce some useful data on the complex organizational problems which I have outlined earlier. If they can enlist the co-operation and support of the community health councils their recommendations will be hard to resist.

How does the future of general practice in the UK appear? In general, the outlook is bright. The prospect is of an increasing number of GPs, a higher proportion of whom will be women, better trained, better equipped, and better supported than their predecessors. What clouds, if any, are there on the horizon? Apart from irritating problems like the persistence of certification for short-term illness, and of difficulties with the payment of related ancillary staff and the notional rent scheme, the largest and darkest cloud must be the constant threat of financial stringency which hangs over the NHS. We in the UK spend less of our national product on health than most other developed nations, and in general receive an excellent deal for our money. If standards are to be maintained, however, and improved in spite of the present climate of economic uncertainty, more money must be found. The levels of remuneration for nurses and all paramedical workers in the community and in hospital have been too low to attract and retain enough first-class people and many of the necessary facilities have been less than adequate. Doctors, especially those who speak English, are a world commodity, and the prospect of integration with the other medical systems within the EEC further increases their potential range.

We shall probably never be able to compete in terms of overall financial reward with some of the wealthiest nations, but we must strive to provide adequate rewards relative to other professions, in the context of a system of payment and organization which engenders professional satisfaction and encourages and supports the GP so that he may give of his best for his patients. In this way we shall provide a basis of high-quality primary medical care in the UK which will stand the NHS in good stead for the next decade and beyond.

REFERENCES

1. Hodgkin, K. (1973). *Towards Earlier Diagnosis* (Edinburgh: E. & S. Livingstone).
2. McWhinney, I. (1964). *The Early Signs of Illness* (London: Pitman Medical Publishing Co.)
3. Fry, J. (1974). *Common Diseases—Their Nature, Incidence and Care* (Lancaster: Medical & Technical Publishing Co.).
4. Cartwright, A. (1967). *Patients and Their Doctors* (London: Routledge and Kegan Paul).
5. Wadsworth, M. E. J., Butterfield, W. J. H., and Blaney, B. (1971). *Health and Sickness. The Choice of Treatment. Perception of Illness and Use of Services in an Urban Community* (London: Tavistock Publications).
6. British Medical Association (1970). *Primary Medical Care.* Planning Unit Report No. 4 (London: BMA).
7. McKeown, T. (1974). *Medicine in Modern Society* (London: Allen and Unwin).

8. ROYAL COLLEGE OF GENERAL PRACTITIONERS (1973). *Present State and Future Needs of General Practice*, third edition (London: RCGP).
9. STEPHEN, W. J. (1974). *Update*, 8, no. 8, 1105–16.
10. COLLINGS, J. S. (1950). *Lancet*, i, 555.
11. HONIGSBAUM, F. (1972). *Jl R. Coll. Gen. Practit.* 172, 22, 429.
12. SMITH, J. WESTON, and MOTTRAM, E. M. (1967). 'Extended use of nursing services in general practice', *Br. med. J.* 4, 672–4.
13. FORMAN, J. A. S., and FAIRBAIRN, E. M. (1968). *Social Casework in General Practice* (Oxford University Press for the Nuffield Provincial Hospitals Trust).
14. GOLDBERG, E. M., NEILL, J., SPEAR, B. M., and FAULKNER, H. C. (1968). 'Social work in general practice', *Lancet*, ii, 552–5.
15. BURR, M. L. and ELWOOD, P. C. (1974). *Update*, 8, no. 7, 988.
16. IRVINE, D. (1972). *Teaching Practices* (London: RCGP).

The future of obstetrics and gynaecology in the National Health Service

IAN CRAFT

IAN CRAFT
FRCS, MRCOG
Obstetrician, Gynaecologist

The future of obstetrics and gynaecology in the National Health Service

Whilst it is apparent that the standard of general health care has markedly improved within this century, this has been particularly the case since the introduction of the NHS. Superficial assessment of care in the field of obstetrics and gynaecology in particular, indicates that steady progress has resulted from consideration of the decline in the maternal mortality and perinatal mortality rates alone. Whilst some may consider that further statistical improvement on the present position is unlikely to be marked, this is probably not the case. Even in recent years there has been increasing concern that the qualitative, as well as the quantitative, aspects of care encompassed by this specialty should improve and, as a result, special attention has been focused upon such subjects as foetal wellbeing during pregnancy and labour and subsequent infant development, besides wider issues such as improving the social status of the family unit by controlling fertility potential, etc. Other specialties have also been concerned with the same general considerations and the resultant greater depth of health care has placed ever-increasing demands on the services and resources of the NHS, which is undergoing the processes of administrative reorganization necessary to deal adequately with this burden. One of the main factors that will determine the extent and need for health care in the future is the reproductive potential of the population and the physiological and pathological consequences that may ensue from human fertility.

A number of factors have been associated with the major improvements in obstetric standards predating the introduction of the NHS and include the introduction of effective antibiotics, blood transfusion facilities, and safer anaesthetic procedures besides the improved welfare status of the community resulting, for example, in a decreasing incidence of pelvic contraction. Some of these same factors also enabled gynaecological practice, especially surgical expertise, to attain new standards, some of which have not been improved upon to this present day. At the same time increasing awareness has been focused upon the need to understand the basic physiology of female reproductive function and its disorders including ovulation, menstruation, pregnancy, and labour. Consequently more consideration has been given to non-surgical sciences such as biochemistry, endocrinology, pharmacology, and physics. More recently clinicians in obstetrics, in particular, have become increasingly aware of the need to recognize situations where the foetus *in utero* is acutely or chronically compromised and a vast array of differing tests of foeto-placental function have been assessed. In gynaecology new therapeutic measures have also resulted in a modification of clinical practice with the availability of synthetic steroids for the treatment of certain disorders of menstruation by non-surgical measures besides providing the most effective reversible method of controlling fertility. Similarly, the introduction of reliable fibroptic systems has enabled the gynaecologist to improve his diagnostic acumen of pelvic disorders besides providing a useful means of performing certain operations. Changes in social pressures have also had particular repercussions on this specialty, especially since the introduction of the Abortion Act in 1967 and with the increasing demand for sterilization procedures for social reasons. There has resulted an alteration in the pattern of gynaecological practice throughout the United Kingdom which has led to changes in the priorities of patients being referred and admitted to hospital for routine gynaecological purposes. It is probable that these social aspects of gynaecology will occupy an increasing proportion of the gynaecologist's time. In obstetrics we can expect greater in-depth management of pregnancy and labour to result in a continuing decrease in maternal and perinatal morbidity and mortality, and greater concern about the issues that might influence the quality of life of both infant and mother. If these then are some of the main topics that are likely to concern the practice of obstetrics and gynaecology, and if this specialty is going to be increasingly concerned with controlling fertility potential of the population, besides endeavouring to ensure that the qualitative and quantitative aspects of obstetric care are optimal, how should it function within the NHS? Before considering these aspects it may be relevant to consider in greater detail the improvements that have occurred and, where valid, critical judgements can be made about the limitations that exist at present.

As a profession we should not be unduly despondent about the future of obstetrics and gynaecology provided adequate resources are made available to administer an efficient service, for enormous strides have occurred in this specialty, which has for too long been considered to be based exclusively on the art of clinical practice rather than on scientific fact. The discovery of sulphonamides in the 1930s and their application into clinical medicine was, for example, associated with a marked reduction in maternal deaths from puerperal sepsis. More recently, the introduction of a variety of tests of foeto-placental function has led to increased foetal salvage. The latter have included serial determinations of plasma or urinary steroid hormones or enzymes reflecting the state of the foeto-placental unit, ultrasound measurements of foetal growth from assessment of increases in the biparietal diameter of the foetal skull, and the use of sophisticated equipment to record variations in the pattern of the foetal heart rate and determinations of the acid base status from analysis of a scalp blood sample. The availability of blood transfusion facilities and the introduction of safer anaesthetic procedures, particularly the more frequent use of regional or epidural, as opposed to general, anaesthesia for operative procedures, besides the use of accessory techniques such as radiological pelvimetry, have all contributed to the improved situation. The routine use of ergometrine at delivery has significantly reduced the incidence of post-partum haemorrhage and the immediate and delayed morbidity that may follow including pituitary insufficiency states. Supplemental oral iron and folic acid administration have decreased the incidence and complications due to megaloblastic and iron-deficiency anaemia states. Similarly, the paediatrician has played an increasing role in recognizing the problems of the premature infant and, by successfully combating alterations in the biochemical, metabolic, and respiratory functions that may result, has in part led to the improvement in the perinatal mortality rate. The importance of contributions made by other disciplines is also apparent; for example, rhesus iso-immunization is now no longer quantitatively the serious problem it was a few years ago since the availability of anti-D immunoglobulin. Even when the disease process does occur, modern obstetric management has mitigated against its serious effects with the introduction of the technique of transfusing the foetus *in utero*. Indeed, perhaps this disease process serves as a good example to illustrate how preventive and therapeutic measures may result in improved obstetric care and how various disciplines may be involved working as a team, including the obstetrician, paediatrician, pathologist, and radiologist, besides valuable ancillary assistance from such sources as the social service department who may need to give advice about providing facilities for the family at home while the patient is in hospital. It is obvious that careful surveillance of patients during pregnancy following their regular attendance at antenatal clinics, continues to have a beneficial effect on obstetric standards by allowing the early recognition of variations from normality and the institution of appropriate measures. The development of rhesus iso-immunization, diabetes mellitus, foetal abnormalities, missed abortion and hydatidiform mole, besides the development of intra-uterine foetal growth retardation and pre-eclampsia, are just some of the conditions that the obstetrician may influence by the institution of early therapeutic measures. On the other hand, whilst improved treatment may have significantly contributed to the decreasing morbidity resulting from such conditions as pre-eclampsia and accidental haemorrhage, this may in part also have been due to a decline in the incidence of these diseases.

A similar improvement in gynaecological care has also evolved but again this has not occurred in isolation. For example, radiotherapy has improved over the last few decades and has been of invaluable benefit in the treatment of certain forms of gynaecological cancer with the consequence that some gynaecologists consider that this is the treatment of choice for certain tumours which would have previously been treated by surgery alone. Combined methods of treatment have also proved of value. In another sphere the understanding of the basic endocrinology of female reproductive function and the availability of synthetic steroid hormones for therapeutic use has altered the rationale and treatment of certain gynaecological disorders by non-surgical means and, on a much broader basis, with the introduction of the contraceptive pill, has resulted in a far more effective and aesthetically acceptablè way of controlling human fertility than was previously possible. The pharmaceutical industry has contributed to the improving standards of both obstetric and gynaecological care following important discoveries so that the effective therapeutic armamentarium now includes antibiotics, oxytocics, ovulatory inhibitors and stimulants, steroids, anti-tumour agents, besides preparations that will control disorders of coagulation. Endoscopic instrumentation has enabled the gynaecologist to establish or confirm rather than presume a given diagnosis and has made it possible to perform various operations by culdoscopy, laparoscopy and, more recently, by hysteroscopy. Besides amendments to surgical technique, improvement in cytology facilities have been of great assistance in diagnosing cervical cancer at an early stage and determining those at risk.

Among the most marked changes in gynaecology in the last few years have been the altered nature of the workload, with more emphasis on social issues such as abortion and sterilization. The increasing demand for termination and the greater awareness of the value of definitive fertility control by sterilization, have placed great stresses on individual departments. Improvements in care have resulted from the introduction of new techniques to deal with both problems, with a resultant decrease in the morbidity that may ensue. For example, we now recognize the advantages of undertaking termination at an early stage in gestation when the amount of cervical trauma necessary to undertake evacuation procedures, is reduced to a minimum thereby minimizing the possible complications of spontaneous miscarriage or premature labour in subsequent pregnancies. Similarly, the introduction of endoscopic sterilization techniques has resulted in a reduced in-patient stay in hospital.

These improving clinical standards do not imply that we should be complacent, for it is apparent at a superficial glance that the standards of clinical care vary markedly throughout the country, suggesting that we have a fragmented rather than a national service. The function of present administration therefore should be that it should recognize the magnitude of problems that exist in obstetrics and gynaecology, both within the hospital service and outside, and be able to view them in the context of total patient care. Effective stable administrative machinery will then be required to administer the manpower and resources that are necessary to deal with the problems and to ensure an efficient service which is sufficiently flexible to allow for changes in the future. The structure of the recently reorganized administration should, in principle, be more efficient at recognizing the inadequacies of medical and nursing manpower facilities and be able to implement appropriate recommendations for the benefit of patient care, always provided that efficient personnel are involved, that the resources are available and that good communications exist.

Although the NHS provides a reasonably good standard of care to the community at large and may be envied as a responsible social service by other countries, there are obviously deficiencies and inadequacies which some may consider to be inherent in the running of any large organization and are analogous to those experienced in administering any large state industry. The most overt and gross problems seen at the grass-roots level are apparent to most clinicians, who find it increasingly difficult to provide an optimum standard of care. One obvious fundamental issue is that central government provides a relatively inadequate proportion of the gross national product for the NHS. It is understandable that many should question the wisdom of not increasing the relative proportions made available for both health and education which are perhaps two of the most important social priorities that exist. If central government is unable to increase the capital resources available, should we dismiss out of hand the possibility that state lotteries could contribute or indeed that the community in each district of the new reorganized NHS should accept some responsibility for the standard of health care provided in its own geographical area? In this latter situation central government could make the provision for a variable involvement depending upon the affluence of any given community.

One of the outstanding problems that beset the NHS is that commerce and industry attract many of the most capable personnel who do not seek employment with the Service because of what appears to be an inadequate remuneration and career structure. Consequently, if the NHS has to rely on the employment of relatively less capable people, especially in ancillary staff positions, it is understandable that failures of communication may result in deficiencies of patient care despite the fact that the responsible senior medical and nursing officers may be of the highest integrity and efficiency. It is therefore to be hoped that the reorganized structure of the NHS will pay particular attention to making occupations within its service particularly attractive.

So far as the distribution of financial resources is concerned within the NHS, it may have been concluded that obstetrics and gynaecology might require a decreasing proportion in relation to other specialties because of the declining birth-rate. This decline, however, does not necessarily imply that the workload will in any way contract, since more detailed management and care are natural consequences of progress. One aspect that has to be considered is who should decide where the priorities exist for distribution of capital resources within obstetrics and gynaecology since there will be increasing costs of all services contributing to patient care and possibly a limitation of available finance. Who, for example, should evaluate whether the expenditure required for stimulating fertility in a very small percentage of the population is out of proportion to that spent on limiting it or indeed for attempting to determine whether congenital or hereditary abnormalities of foetal development exist, in time for definitive action? Similarly, one might ask, should central administration have any influence over the cost and range of pharmaceutical preparations; if so, how should this be effected since expenditure on these preparations is very large? It is to be hoped that the reorganized administration will be more efficient in ensuring that such funds as are available will be distributed fairly to the different regional, area, and district authorities depending on relative needs, and will not be duplicated or wasted in the future, thereby preventing the exacerbation of an already deteriorating position.

So far as medical politics are concerned, it is a fact that one of the most contentious worries of clinicians is that recommendations made as a result of local divisional meetings may not be given a proper and sympathetic assessment by higher administrators who may no longer have a clinical orientation. Some feel, therefore, that representative bodies such as the Royal College of Obstetricians and Gynaecologists and associations of professional doctors, besides the Royal College of Midwives, should have easy access to those concerned with over-all policy at a high level. The need for such interchange is apparent if one alone considers the inadequacies of the implementation of the Abortion Act within the framework of the NHS. There is also concern that the new administration should ensure that there is better integration between the hospital and community, possibly by arranging meetings and symposia at district general and teaching hospitals for the benefit of medical, nursing, and other personnel, from within the hospital service and outside in the community. Besides focusing attention on the specific needs of obstetrics and gynaecology in a given geographical area, it may in particular lead to good relations between GPs and hospital staff and perhaps offset the already declining involvement of GPs in practical obstetrics, besides ensuring that the standards of hospital care are maintained and improved.

If we now turn our attention to the distribution of capital resources, it is apparent that previously it has been difficult to proportion these to the relative needs of specific areas, partly because of the political influences of central government but also because of political influences that exist within the framework of medical practice, involving opinions of doctors in the DHSS and in teaching and peripheral hospitals. As a result a regional, as opposed to a national, health service has come to exist with marked differences in the standards of care provided. If we just consider the differences in the complement of medical personnel of all grades in hospitals undertaking the same workload, for example, the same number of deliveries and gynaecological operations per year, marked differences will be found to occur throughout the United Kingdom. Who then should be surprised if inadequacies of medical attention should result? A decline in medical standards is a natural outcome if there is poor supervision or tuition of the staff, lack of continuity of care because of reliance on frequent *locum tenens* appointments or because of inadequate attention being paid to individual patients as a result of excessive workloads experienced by doctors working in certain areas. The new framework of organization of the NHS should bring to the attention of those dealing with medical manpower, the need of increasing or redistributing available personnel.

If now we consider the medical staff structure in the hospital service in a little more detail it is obvious that the situation is not perfect. Why, it might be asked, in a service apparently envied by the world, are more than half the hospital appointments, up to and including senior registrar status, occupied by graduates from medical schools from outside the United Kingdom? It is true that this in part reflects the entry of graduates to study for higher examinations and diplomas and to gain theoretical and practical experience, but where are all the indigenous graduates of our own medical schools, who on theoretical grounds alone, should have been able to occupy such positions and why are they not in the hospital service? Several factors are probably responsible, including inadequate forward planning and relatively poor remuneration compared with practitioners in other spheres at home and overseas and possibly even a lack of significant differential from other members in the community who have not had to study for many years. It is also apparent from a junior hospital doctor's point of view that a planned specialization programme occurring over a definitive period of time with obvious outlets after attainment of specialization would have advantages and would retain many who at the present moment leave the hospital service. Many junior doctors also feel dissatisfied that their career prospects are still subject to the patronage of some senior colleagues and that their appointments are not integrated in any definite manner either in their nature or in location. It is likely that the provision of rotational and research appointments within the framework of postgraduate education would offer a stimulus to training.

These sort of considerations may make hospital specialization a more attractive prospect but there is still concern that the specialty of obstetrics and gynaecology in particular is ceasing to attract sufficient numbers of capable graduates. Besides the general considerations mentioned, it is probable that the nature of the work, including long hours of duty and the recent tendency of gynaecology to be particularly concerned with social issues such as abortion, contraception, and sterilization, and less with the art of surgery, may be responsible. If indeed these are relevant facts, how can the NHS ensure that this tendency will be ameliorated or rectified? Or course, some of these concepts apply equally to the recruitment of nursing staff in obstetrics and gynaecology since therapeutic abortion may be offensive, especially when nurses are personally involved in the operating suite or on the ward where a therapeutic mid-trimester termination is induced. In addition, the recent emergence of nursing agency organizations without any statutory standards of efficiency, remunerating their staff at higher levels compared with the NHS employees, has understandably led to discord and serves to highlight just one injustice of the present position. This anomaly can only be solved by remunerating nursing staff adequately and by ensuring that a nursing career is fulfilling, for by so doing this will eliminate the reported differing standards and lack of continuity of patient care that have arisen in some situations. Similarly, whilst it is not an inherent fault of the structure of the NHS organization, it is important to recognize the role of midwives in particular, since there is increasing concern in their midst that they are less involved in the traditional considerations of care of the mother throughout the antenatal period and delivery of her child, and more concerned with the supervision of monitoring apparatus, recording uterine activity and foetal heart rate patterns, now commonly found on labour wards. In addition, while appreciating the benefits that may ensue from epidural analgesia, they are critical if an operative delivery is more likely to result, thereby eliminating their traditional role. Is it possible that in the future the Royal College of Midwives and the Royal College of Obstetricians and Gynaecologists, will sanction greater midwife involvement in practical obstetrical procedures such as uncomplicated forceps delivery and the like, thereby ensuring that midwives' attention is an integral part of total patient care without of necessity diminishing the doctor's role? One might also consider whether the training of already sophisticated staff nurses in the practice of midwifery would be made more attractive and result in more remaining within the specialty if many of the mundane and routine chores associated with the antenatal and post-natal management of patients, was dealt with by alternative personnel. There are other stresses under which midwives function including alterations in the workload that result from changes in a variety of medical policies. One such example is the increased nursing involvement that results from the introduction of more liberal indications for induction of labour and the wider acceptance of active management of labour with stimulation of uterine activity using various oxytocics, including oxytocin and prostaglandins, administered by differing routes that require careful and detailed management to ensure that the foetus and mother are not jeopardized. The problems of this increasing workload and the relative limitations of the nursing resources may be best brought to everyone's attention at divisional Cogwheel meetings and as a result there may be a revision of codes of practice within given departments. There is little doubt that the institution of divisional meetings has greatly facilitated highlighting deficiencies in the running of departments of obstetrics and gynaecology and led to appropriate consideration of priorities. There is also concern, however, that not all administrative changes have of necessity been beneficial since nursing standards may deteriorate following the promotion of some staff to administrative positions which they would otherwise not have wished to occupy before the introduction of the Salmon recommendations. On the other hand it is likely that benefits will accrue from both nursing and medical staff being able to attend courses relating to the administration of the NHS.

Another general question to be asked is whether we are adequately training undergraduates in this specialty in the light of changing patterns of obstetrics and gynaecology? From a superficial glance one would expect that greater emphasis should be given to social issues such as population control, the quality of life, and the like. However it is not only with the education of prospective doctors that we should be concerned but also with their predecessors. There is much to commend a more comprehensive community health education programme directed predominantly at school education for we cannot expect future generations to consider such aspects as the need and methods of fertility control; the hazards of 'permissiveness' including the increasing incidence of venereal disease; the effects of environmental factors including diet, smoking, and drugs on general health and pregnancy in particular; and of preventive measures such as cytological screening for cervical cancer, if the present generation of doctors and educationists is not predominantly concerned with these issues. It is also to be hoped that senior personnel in the DHSS should be anxious to bring to the attention of the public the values of educating future generations in this manner. Whilst many appreciate the wisdom of drawing attention to the disadvantages of smoking, similar campaigns, particularly into some of the issues described previously, could be promoted as issues of special social importance by making available information in written, spoken, and visual form in education centres and outside, even utilizing the facilities of the press, radio, and television. For example, it may seem odd to many that in view of the particular problems that presently confront us with regard to population control, such important topics as contraception are rarely seen on television and when they are they are usually screened on a minority channel and at a time when they are seen by a relatively selective audience who is least at risk. Of course audiovisual aids are of particular value in providing educational information not only to the public in general but to doctors and midwives in particular, and there are advantages in having clearly presented topics available for distribution from such central authorities as teaching or district hospital libraries or the Royal College of Obstetricians and Gynaecologists and the Royal College of Midwives.

If we now consider the standards of obstetric and gynaecological care from the patients' point of view, it is apparent that there are inadequacies which vary in different regions despite a general improvement in the standard of care. In some situations the indications for a hospital confinement are much more stringent than others, even for women expecting their first baby, because of a limited availability of hospital beds, so that in some areas in the northern counties of England, a large percentage of deliveries may be carried out in GP units unattached to the hospital obstetric department, whereas in other more favoured situations the suggested ideal of having 100 per cent hospital confinement may nearly exist. Similarly, it is apparent that there is uneven distribution of facilities for performing laboratory and monitoring investigations that some consider should be readily available for all obstetric and gynaecology departments throughout the country. For example, even at this present time, ultrasound facilities exist in relatively few centres. Other complaints that are commonly aired include the delays that patients experience before being seen by a medical practitioner, and the delays that result before even minor gynaecological procedures can be performed. Conflicting medical advice obviously leads to dissatisfaction, especially if it is apparent that there are different medical criteria for considering, for example, requests for therapeutic abortion and sterilization. Whilst it is understandable that there should be different subjective assessments about the indications for these procedures compared with opinions relating to organic disorders, they nevertheless relate to deep emotive and personal feelings experienced by the patient. On a more general note it is distressing that successive governments have had to restrict capital expenditure on new hospital buildings and available funds for research which may be seen in the eyes of the public as reflecting non-optimal standards of comfort and a slowing-down of the natural evolution of improvements in the standards of the clinical sciences and care that they have come to expect to receive.

Future obstetric care

It is the writer's firm opinion that, so far as future obstetric practice is concerned, all confinements should ideally occur within hospital departments. That is not to say that deliveries at home or in a small GP unit unattached to hospital departments of obstetrics and gynaecology do not provide a valuable service at present, or that the surrounding environment is not better as far as the patient is concerned, appearing more humanitarian and less clinical. Nevertheless, without doubt, there is value in trying to achieve a 100 per cent hospital confinement rate essentially for the benefit of the patient since all the necessary facilities are likely to be available should assistance or interference be required, with a resulting reduction in the perinatal mortality rate. Besides this consideration it is also likely that the provisions that need to be made for an extensive emergency obstetric flying squad service could be reduced. Provided hospital authorities recognize the value placed by patients on their home comforts including having their husbands in attendance at delivery, besides the introduction of more liberal visiting for relatives, then such a policy is likely to gain public acceptance, especially if the staff situation improves allowing increasing personal attention. Even if the staffing situation does not markedly alter in the foreseeable future there must be a greater awareness on the part of obstetric nurses and doctors that personal considerations are of vital importance and that undue reliance and attention should not be given to the ever-increasing array of instrumentation that is used during labour and delivery to the exclusion of humanitarian patient care. There is little wonder that some now feel that 'it is the machines that are having the babies'. Within the precincts of the hospital department, obstetric care can be achieved by both midwives, GPs, or hospital specialist staff acting in harmony and without discord or loss of personal involvement, and yet always knowing that facilities of the hospital department are available to deal with complications, for example, in patients whose obstetric care is being supervised by their GP using the hospital facilities. Whilst some may consider that all deliveries should be under the supervision of the specialist hospital staff, this would mean that some excellent GPs would be denied the opportunity of participating in obstetric management. Such a decision, however, should be unnecessary provided good communications exist between GPs and hospital staff so that immediate consultation is sought should any type of problem arise. So far as antenatal care is concerned, there is no need to suggest that great changes should occur in the system of management, with provisions of 'shared care' between hospital and GPs still being a feature of the surveillance of uncomplicated pregnancies. Of course, in some areas it will take a considerable time before the suggested ideal of all confinements occurring in hospital is achieved and in the meantime other possibilities should be considered; for example, attempts could be made to deliver increasing numbers of patients in hospital obstetric units by expanding labour ward staff and increasing the involvement of the community services including a temporary expansion of district midwifery facilities sufficient to enable them to cope with the discharge of the majority of fit and suitable mothers to their home environment; for example, within twenty-four hours of delivery. Even now a varied pattern of the time of discharge of normal mothers from hospital from two to ten days exists in different areas depending upon the bed availability and the workload. Even in situations where there is not a shortage of hospital beds it is quite probable that many healthy mothers would prefer to be discharged much earlier than is normally the case, especially multigravidae, but at the present time such provision is limited by the availability of supervisory district midwives. The introduction of such a flexible service will almost certainly lead to an improvement in standards of care and a reduction in over-all costs.

It is also to be hoped that the new administration will assist with the improvement in standards of care by recognizing the limitations alluded to previously. Surely it is not too much to hope that every district general hospital will have such essential services as an ultrasound department giving valuable assistance for the determination of foetal growth-rate, foetal abnormalities, and localization of the placenta, besides being of use in other spheres? Similarly, every clinician should have available to his department the laboratory investigations that are necessary to indicate that foetal-placental function is satisfactory, such as urinary steroid hormone determinations, although in the future it is to be hoped that new, simple, accurate, and reliable indices will be found which will indicate foetal wellbeing from analysis of a random plasma sample. One of the present limitations of assessing sex steroid hormone concentrations in either plasma or urine samples, even using radio-immuno-assay techniques, is the fact that serial samples are necessary if they are to serve as prognostic indices. In the future more and more stress is likely to be placed upon detecting specific foetal abnormalities *in utero* in the mid-trimester of pregnancy following examination of amniotic fluid samples using biochemical and chromosomal techniques at a time when therapeutic abortion could still be achieved if desired. Initially such investigations are likely to be available only at specific regional centres; for example, for the determination of alpha-foeto-protein to exclude central nervous system malformations and chromosome analysis for mongolism. It is also likely that an increasing spectrum of investigations will be performed upon the maternal blood sample taken at the time of the first attendance at hospital, which at present is analysed for haemoglobin concentration, blood group factors, the presence of sickling, rubella antibody titre, evidence of past or previous venereal disease and Australia antigen. Provided adequate provisions are made for supporting future research from such bodies as the DHSS, the MRC, industrial companies, and charitable trusts, then there is hope that the prediction of certain abnormalities may become possible from simple laboratory tests. For example, is it too much to hope that in the future it will be possible to predict the likelihood of patients developing pre-eclampsia or intra-uterine foetal growth retardation from a simple plasma sample? Is it also too much to hope that effective measures will be developed to deal with some of these problems, much in the same manner as has resulted in the treatment of rhesus iso-immunization? Since there is an increasing awareness of the quality of 'survivors' there is also much to commend effective educational material being made available to prospective parents, either presented in printed form or audio-visually at special meetings, stressing the importance of environmental factors in health, including diet, smoking, and drugs, and explaining clearly in outline the physiology of pregnancy and labour and early infant development. The only problem relating to this aspect of care is that those usually most at risk are those least likely to take advantage of the information. Hence the earlier stress placed on the need to educate the young.

So far as practical obstetrical management is concerned, there is little effective therapeutic treatment other than bed rest that can at present be offered to patients in the last trimester who have, for example, intra-uterine foetal growth retardation, but it is not beyond the bounds of possibility that intra-uterine feeding may become a distinct reality. It is only recently that more rational management of certain problems is now possible following the introduction of such facilities as performing lecithin sphingomyelin ratios on amniotic fluid as indicators of the likely development of the respiratory distress syndrome. Extension of this practice throughout the country and future developments in this field are likely to be of value since they indicate the most logical way of achieving delivery before term, if this becomes essential, and may serve as an indicator that treatment with adrenal steroids will be useful. It is also quite possible that further advances will occur with the development of finer fibroptic systems allowing the use of inspection of the foetus *in utero* by the practice of foetoscopy to exclude significant foetal abnormalities and to allow accurate intra-uterine transfusion where this is desired.

The discovery of new drugs may markedly affect future obstetric management in many ways as exemplified by the recent applications of prostaglandins in this field. The previous conservative approach to an intra-uterine foetal death is now no longer justifiable, knowing how effective prostaglandins are following their administration, particularly by the extra-amniotic route in this instance. Whilst oxytocin is relatively inefficient in the mid-trimester of pregnancy when a hydatidiform mole may be present, prostaglandins are likely to be much more effective. It is also quite likely that newer oxytocics will be found which may be even better than prostaglandins and that other compounds may be developed which have specific properties for potential use such as dilating placental blood vessels. The latter would be of particular value in the treatment of pre-eclampsia and the small-for-dates syndrome. Now that planned delivery is more often associated with the use of oxytocic preparations, stress tests are being more extensively used to assess the foetus at risk who is unlikely to stand the stress of labour and it is probable that other simple, safe, and reliable tests will be developed.

Although it is only recently that obstetricians and midwives have in general come to consider the value of having standard induction policies, such as the use of forewater rupture combined with intravenous oxytocin titration, there is much to commend a flexible and selective approach. Patients who have unfavourable induction features as assessed on pelvic examination, are generally in labour a relatively long time and require quantitatively greater amounts of oxytocic than those in whom the features are particularly favourable. Whilst intravenous oxytocics are rational for the former group, more simple measures, such as oral prostaglandin therapy, may be particularly useful in the latter, especially in the multigravida and allow maximum midwifery involvement to be given to those most at risk. Whilst there are advantages from an organizational point of view in having active and selective policies for the induction and acceleration of labour, providing what many would consider to be 'daylight obstetrics', inherent problems in administration are likely to result if inadequate staff are available. Also caution should be exercised to prevent the induction-delivery interval from becoming the 'be all' and 'end all' of obstetric excellence since without doubt each woman must have an inherent optimum oxytocic responsiveness at any stage of gestation which may vary with time and which exogenous oxytocic administration may prejudice. Is it too much to hope that we shall develop an 'indicator' which will ensure that optimum myometrial responsiveness results from exogenous oxytocic therapy or endogenous oxytocin or prostaglandin release? Whilst modern technology has provided us with sophisticated equipment to administer these drugs, such as infusion pumps, some with safety feedback mechanisms incorporating recording of uterine pressure and activity from an intra-uterine pressure catheter, future developments are likely to result in more portable and simplified equipment being made available for routine care in all units rather than in specialized centres. Again it is probable that in the future, provision will be made for recording uterine activity and the foetal heart rate continuously throughout labour from channels in every labour ward with a console panel present in the administrative centre of the labour ward suite. Although facilities for performing acid-base determinations of foetal blood samples have become increasingly available throughout the country, it is also to be hoped that it will be possible to equip all obstetric departments with monitoring apparatus that records the uterine activity and the foetal heart rate and that simple methods will be found to predict which variations in the foetal heart rate pattern are of clinical significance and which are not, thereby indicating the need for operative interference. Research should also be focused upon the possibility of developing a non-invasive technique which will continuously indicate the wellbeing of the foetus *in utero*. Future developments in paediatric care will also parallel those in obstetrics and will lead to an over-all improvement in results.

Future gynaecological care

Similar stresses to those caused in obstetrics by having liberal induction policies have resulted from the workload caused by the implementation of the Abortion Act, since it is apparent that the NHS structure is grossly inadequate to deal with this particular problem. In certain areas abortion is difficult to obtain even when genuine grounds exist, either because of the unsympathetic attitude of certain gynaecologists or GPs or because of delays before referral for an opinion, or because of the extreme pressure of work within the hospital departments of gynaecology, and it remains a fact that private practice and charitable organizations deal with many thousands of abortions that should be the responsibility of the NHS. Whilst it is to be hoped that in the future expansion of contraception services will result in a reduction in the request for abortion, this does not necessarily follow. Whatever recent judgements have been made into the workings of the Abortion Act, it is the opinion of many clinicians that there are gross limitations in the implementation of the service and extensive repercussions affecting routine gynaecological practice. Perhaps part of the problem stems from the way the Abortion Act was drawn up, allowing termination on grounds so variable as to be construed in different manners by different gynaecologists. In some areas abortion is almost 'on-demand' and in others it is extremely difficult to obtain and this divergence is surely basically wrong for opposing judgements may be passed on a given individual or on different individuals having the same grounds. It is possible that some of the confusion that now exists would be eliminated either by more strictly limiting the grounds for termination of pregnancy or by making it legally 'on-demand', but, it seems likely that public awareness of the issues at stake will not now allow for more restriction. The prospect of abortion 'on-demand' may or may not aggravate the practical problems that presently exist but this concept raises other issues. Who, for example, would perform these procedures and where? There are those who feel that special clinics run by the DHSS and manned by well-trained and well-remunerated personnel, should be set up either attached to a hospital department of gynaecology or situated outside. This would at least allow routine gynaecological practice to revert to its traditional role and would eliminate the need for charitable organizations to exist, although there may be advantages in utilizing the resources of such organizations within the framework of the NHS. One obvious total inadequacy of leaving the situation as it is at present is that all too often there is a poor follow-up and yet, as a profession, we should be particularly concerned about evaluating the psychological and physical effects of abortion and be anxious to improve techniques so that the chances of undesirable sequelae occurring are minimised or prevented.

So far as techniques are concerned, there would be advantages in extending the out-patient abortion services that have been started in some centres, especially if the service is to remain within the confines of hospital departments of gynaecology, but the efficiency of very early suction procedures depends upon the time of referral to hospital by the patient's GP. It is quite likely that there will be great improvements in the techniques used to terminate pregnancies, especially by non-surgical means and these could result in dramatic alterations in the need to involve existing hospital facilities. It is possible, for example, that effective synthetic or naturally occurring anti-fertility agents will be found which will induce luteolysis or act by some other mechanism and will eventually become freely available so that susceptible women may control their own fertility destiny. On theoretical grounds there would be much to commend the availability of a simple, safe, and effective agent preferably taken orally, which would induce menstruation that had been delayed for a few days in women who had been exposed to the possible risk of pregnancy, and yet be free of any significant influence in impairing ovulation in subsequent cycles. Whilst the present generation of clinicians may consider this concept of controlling human fertility to be revolutionary, and be worried that aspects of patient care currently being supervised by gynaecologists will be eroded, it is quite feasible that this will become a reality. The introduction of these methods would influence the need for special termination clinics and their staff structure which is yet another argument for ensuring that the administration of the NHS needs to be sufficiently flexible to deal with such modification of treatment.

Whilst the NHS has accepted responsibility for contraception, it is a fact that no co-ordinated scheme exists for integrating this aspect of health care throughout the United Kingdom, since GPs, gynaecologists, and charitable organizations all play a role, each in a dissimilar location. There would be much to commend a central administrative structure dealing, for example, with either this aspect alone or with the wider issue of controlling fertility, including therapeutic abortion and sterilization procedures performed upon both the male and female. Similarly, on a practical level there would be advantages in utilizing specific facilities known to the public where advice could always be obtained. The gynaecological out-patient departments of district general hospitals would serve as ideal locations for clinics, especially in the evenings when the departments are unoccupied and could be staffed by responsible doctors who have a specific interest in this subject, whether employees of the hospital service or GPs. It might be considered that a hospital location has some advantages over the alternative possibility of having contraception facilities available in the expanding health centres since the advice offered allows a certain anonymity for those who prefer this and yet allows free access to other hospital facilities, such as for detecting venereal disease, which is an ever-increasing problem. Similarly, referral to other departments following the detection of associated disorders, such as breast lumps and gynaecological abnormalities, would also be possible. On the other hand this idea may be impractical in certain rural areas where the population is sparsely distributed. In these situations, advice may be most effectively given either by the GP or by other community personnel trained in contraception, visiting the home. A flexible administration could achieve this end.

Since gynaecological waiting-lists have become even longer because of increasing abortion demands, more attention has been given to performing minor gynaecological procedures, including abortion, on an out-patient basis often under local anaesthesia, and such a trend is likely to continue and be extended. Cervical erosions treated by low-heat coagulation or cryosurgery, and out-patient curettage and salpingography, have obvious benefits in eliminating the need for bed availability and ensuring that more serious disorders get priority admission. Extra resources should be available for expansion of this service in certain areas whilst the problem of long waiting-lists remains.

With regard to sterilization of the female, this practice is being increasingly performed by diathermy coagulation at laparoscopy. Occlusive clips are likely to gain wider acceptance in the future following application by laparoscopy since less tissue damage will result, and accidental burns will be eliminated. In addition, should reversibility be required, re-establishment of tubal continuity will be a more feasible proposition. Other improvements are also likely to result; for example, compounds will probably be found which will cause proximal tubal occlusion following a simple injection of a solution through the cervix although as yet none so far tried has been found to be ideal. One of the disadvantages of this latter approach is that it is unlikely that reversibility will be easy to accomplish. It is to be hoped that other potentially reversible techniques will become available for application to both men and women. Since gynaecology should be concerned about total fertility potential, it may be relevant that gynaecologists should be more involved with the practice of vasectomy since this does not necessarily fall within the domain of either the urologist or general surgeon. A similar situation analogous to that arising following the introduction of the Abortion Act now exists in hospital departments of surgery since they are unable to cope with the requests for vasectomy to be performed within the NHS. Consequently, most GPs refer patients for these procedures to charitable organizations, often the same organization that is concerned with abortion and contraception. Once again there would be advantages in having some central administrative structure particularly concerned with this issue since there is no factual information on how many vasectomies have been performed in recent years or on what the future needs might be. The advantages of introducing an effective service placed in existing hospital facilities such as out-patient departments and out-patient operating theatres, at times when they are not otherwise occupied, is that they would allow effective counselling, and the operations and post-operative management could be conducted within the confines of one location. The back-up services of the pathology department would enable the medico-legal requirements of negative semen counts to be performed and also make available referral opinion should complications arise.

One of the natural consequences of the community being more concerned about fertility control is that infertility has become a relatively more important subject since fewer babies are available for adoption. Recent advances in pharmacology that have allowed previously infertile women to become pregnant, because of the use of agents stimulating the pituitary-ovarian axis, will be extended in the future with the isolation, synthesis, and application of hypothalamic releasing factors, and more sophisticated control of these processes will presumably make multiple births less likely to result.

On another front other therapeutic compounds are likely to gain increasingly in the management of cancer which is well exemplified by the excellent progress that has resulted in the treatment of chorion carcinoma. Although some clinicians may feel concerned about the advisability of special centres being developed to deal with genital cancer, their introduction is likely to improve standards of patient care since those in any such centre should be able to benefit from the expertise made available from continuing advances in immunology, radiology, radiotherapy, surgery, and therapeutics. Careful documentation and registration of case-records of patients with various types of cancer, ideally utilizing computerized data, should have advantages for assessment of various methods of treatment. Such prerequisites should be of great value in the management of all patients treated in the field of obstetrics and gynaecology for at the present moment retrieval of factual information from case-records is far too difficult and inaccurate.

Whilst the value of cytological screening for cervical cancer is already available throughout the United Kingdom, too few of those at risk avail themselves of this service and further public motivation is required to ensure that regular cervical smears are taken throughout life and not just in isolation as at present. Cervical smears could be taken on every patient at her first attendance at hospital in each pregnancy, and at contraception clinics ideally situated within the hospital as suggested previously. With central records available in any given district, this should contribute to reducing the potential of cervical cancer developing and recognizing those at risk. It is understandable that many in our community are not keen on the idea of having central registers recording details of the health care of individuals within a given community but one has only to appreciate the standards of improvement in care that have resulted in some communities where this is practised to realize the marked benefits that may accrue. As gynaecologists we should also be concerned about other aspects of health care in general since it would seem illogical to be particularly motivated towards performing cervical smears for the early detection of cervical cancer and yet be unconcerned about the need to perform chest X-rays on the ever-increasing numbers of women who now smoke heavily and who as a consequence have an increased risk of developing lung cancer. Finally, perhaps one other aspect that gynaecologists will become increasingly concerned with in the future will be the management of post-menopausal women, not specifically with derangements commonly associated with this age-group, for example utero-vaginal prolapse, but more with the general question of health care that appertains to depletion of endogenous sex steroid hormone levels particularly of ovarian origin. It is to be hoped in the future that specific research will indicate which women in particular will be most likely to develop this problem, so that simple, additive hormonal therapy can be given at an early stage to minimize the development of conditions known to be associated with oestrogen deficiency, such as osteoporosis and cerebral and cardiovascular manifestations. Whilst the span of life may not necessarily be prolonged in such patients, the quality may be improved by administration of small amounts of steroids, possibly given indefinitely.

In conclusion whilst we should reflect on the improvements that have resulted in greater health care in general, and in obstetrics and gynaecology in particular, especially since the introduction of the NHS, we should be increasingly motivated to rectify some of the faults that have been outlined. Is it too much to hope that increased capital resources will be made available by central government to the NHS, allowing the practice of integrated community and hospital medicine in modern buildings, staffed by adequate personnel of all types and grades, whose employment is rewarding and associated with fair remuneration and a clear career structure, supervised by efficient administration which would allow for a steady improvement in the standard of clinical sciences and consequently of patient care, which was forseen by those who introduced the service almost four decades ago? The public are likely to answer 'no'.

Epidemiology, health, and health services

TOM MEADE

TOM MEADE
BM, MRCP
Epidemiologist

Epidemiology, health, and health services

'If, for the next twenty years no further research were to be carried out, if there were a moratorium on research, the application of what is already known, of what has already been discovered, would result in widespread improvement in world health.'

The brief article ('Health in the world of to-morrow') in which these words appeared was an abstract of Lord Rosenheim's address to the Regional Committee for Europe of the World Health Organization, on the occasion of WHO's twentieth anniversary (38). The paper gives a simple, direct account of medicine's achievements, failures, and future challenges, an apt starting-point for anyone concerned, whether in 'the under-doctored disease-ridden bush of developing countries, or in the urban areas of our so-called civilized countries'. But the address contained another, less often quoted sentence: 'It must increasingly be the purpose of the medical profession, and of all who work with them, to aim at prevention rather than cure.'

The epidemiologist's potential contribution is largely encompassed by these two principles, though they create something of an apparent paradox. For the application of knowledge in health care calls for the synthesis into a workable service of information usually obtained from varying sources and by different methods; it is not primarily concerned with the more basic aspects of the issue, the now seemingly distant means to a present end. On the other hand, prevention of many of the world's major diseases depends on an apparently quite different approach—the fragmentation of the problem into its component parts, and the detailed study of each by whatever means are necessary; here, continued technological development will increasingly be a prerequisite. The social scientist and the operational research worker are the epidemiologist's colleagues in the first instance, the haematologist and the biochemist in the second—and the clinician, of course, throughout. Figure 1 illustrates the interlocking nature of modern epidemiology; the scheme has general applicability, though it is exemplified by two major health issues of our time: the consequences of cigarette smoking, and the prevention of clinical arterial disease, especially ischaemic heart disease (IHD). Because epidemiology is so closely concerned with prevention, it has hitherto found its main use in studies of causation. For example, the observational studies of Doll and Hill (15, 16) on the consequences of smoking, and Hill's (22) guidelines for assessing the likelihood of a causal relationship, especially in situations where experiment is not possible, are milestones in modern epidemiology. But why do some smokers develop lung cancer, and others avoid it? What 'causes' cigarette smoking in the first place? Why has it proved so difficult to modify smoking habits? These questions only have to be asked to make it clear that both the epidemiologist and the social scientist can each (at least in theory) contribute to the several separate stages of inquiry, aetiological or preventive, that the problem demands.

Equally, the epidemiologist can approach the causation of arterial disease by asking (with the biochemist, the haematologist, and the pathologist) whether lipid infiltration, thrombosis, or some other process is the main cause of atheroma, and what the relationship really is between pathological changes and clinical disease; or by trying to identify environmental circumstances and personal habits associated with the disease—this is, perhaps, an area in which he is often self-sufficient; or by joining with the social scientist in attempting to clarify and perhaps modify some of the social features he believes responsible for the disease.

Often, discovery of the cause of a disease is sufficient to prevent it; publicity about thalidomide saw the virtual end of the phocomelia associated with its use in pregnancy (though the whole episode lasted longer than one would like to believe possible now). But where association may still not be accepted as implying causation, experimental epidemiology, or intervention, may be the next step. The association demonstrated between cigarette smoking and lung cancer, including the diminishing risks in ex-smokers, was so clear that trials to strengthen it would have been

CAUSATION ⇄	INTERVENTION* →	IMPLEMENTATION and EVALUATION
Smoking		
(i) 'Causes' of smoking itself.	Not much used except in multi-factor intervention trials of ischaemic heart disease (see below).	(i) How can smokers be encouraged to stop?
(ii) Association of smoking with various diseases.		(ii) Can children be encouraged/made not to start?
(iii) Which smokers develop smoking related diseases?		(iii) Use of economic measures in reducing smoking.
		(iv) Introduction of safer smoking methods and habits.
		(v) Possible screening for smokers at especially high risk.
Ischaemic heart disease		
(i) Personal habits and environmental associations.	Trials of dietary measures, clofibrate, hypotensive agents, etc., in prevention; of place of treatment for myocardial infarction, etc.	(i) Some countries formally recommend 'prudent' diet.
(ii) Disordered function, for example 'hypercoagulability', hyperlipidaemia, hypertension.		(ii) Treatment of severe hypertension prevents cerebrovascular disease; position over ischaemic heart disease not yet clear. ?Introduce screening for hypertension.
(iii) Causes of atheroma; relationship of atheroma to clinical disease.		

*Intervention gives information about causes as well as suggesting methods of prevention, treatment, etc.

FIG. 1. The stages of epidemiological inquiry, exemplified by some aspects of cigarette smoking and of ischaemic heart disease.

unethical—and virtually impracticable (though, surprisingly, the difficulties of providing incontrovertible evidence about some of the effects of smoking can still [35] be overlooked). For arterial disease, on the other hand, intervention studies are now an accepted and essential part of its epidemiological study, being used to investigate both causation and the possibilities for prevention. For certain aspects of some diseases, experimental studies may be an appropriate starting-point, even in the absence of a very clear picture of their causes. The introduction of mammography for the investigation of breast tumours carried obvious theoretical potential for the early diagnosis of malignant disease; trials now suggest (64) that early treatment following its use may result in a reduction of breast cancer mortality in women over the age of about 50. At this intervention stage, it becomes necessary for several disciplines to consider jointly the practicalities of a possible future service: who needs it, whether and how it should be provided, how much it will cost, and so on.

Finally, epidemiology finds obvious immediate applications in studies of needs and demands for health services and of their effectiveness; it is here particularly, though not exclusively, that the epidemiologist carries out his research with the economist, the sociologist, and the operational researcher, and perhaps also works with the manager and administrator in implementing his findings. But it is clear that at any stage, from aetiological study to implementation in practice, today's epidemiologist is likely to associate closely with those in many other disciplines.

This view of the uses of epidemiology (34) is widely accepted (though some still tend to limit interpretation of the subject to studies of aetiology and perhaps of prevention); it is the starting-point for the undisputed importance of epidemiology as the community physician's basic method, and has several important implications.

First, the earlier paradox is more apparent than real; both the provision of health care and the prevention of disease may lead the epidemiologist into collaboration with the laboratory scientist, the social scientist, or the community physician and his colleagues. The mutual suspicions with which different groups in social medicine have often tended to view one another, and which various aspects of the birth of community medicine accentuated, are, like labour pains, real and probably inevitable, but hopefully the prelude to something more positive. This is not, however, to deny that there are difficulties associated with effective interdisciplinary work (some are discussed later), or that there may be something of a cult about the 'multidisciplinary team', often established, one suspects, for its own sake.

Secondly, who is an epidemiologist? Epidemiology is based on the study of groups or populations; strictly, it implies nothing essentially medical (nor, specifically, anything to do with infection) though by usage it is the population-based study of health and disease. The basis of the subject is really no more than a logical, ordered method of collecting and interpreting mainly numerical data. Consequently, anyone working with these kinds of data, and concerned with issues of health and disease in human population groups, is using epidemiological methods, even if he does not call himself an epidemiologist. Thirdly, the terminological convention by which 'health services research' tends to replace 'epidemiology' the moment some immediate application can be perceived, is unhelpful. Epidemiology is population-based research and development, whether the cause of stomach cancer or the effectiveness of home nursing is at issue.

Finally, as the result of its successes so far and of its potential in the future, epidemiology has been propelled over a very few years into a position of unprecedented and still largely unrecognized influence. Much clinical research, as well as environmental medicine, disease prevention, and most facets of community medicine, depend on population-based study methods. It is increasingly likely that the clinical research worker, for example, trying to compare different treatments for a disease, or to measure what he is actually achieving, will be put in touch with the epidemiologist, at least for advice, and quite possibly with a view to joint studies. It is not hard to see that almost any aspect of modern medicine, curing, caring, or preventive, is open to epidemiological study, especially where its effectiveness is concerned.

This state of affairs carries its dangers, also. First, there are some areas where the epidemiological approach, though possible, is not the most appropriate, and insistence otherwise may actually hinder progress. The epidemiologist, as well as others concerned, has to be able to identify these instances. Secondly, the epidemiologist runs the risk of appearing a knowall or busybody, a view undoubtedly held by some, and not always without justification.

He certainly is in an excellent position to have an over-all, synoptic view of medicine, but a significant epidemiological contribution increasingly entails a mastery of the specific technicalities of the subject concerned, and, given the growing tendency towards specialization within population-based research, it is unlikely that more than a very few epidemiologists will be able to be jacks of all trades. Furthermore, effective collaboration means that the epidemiologist has to be aware of the real but sometimes improbable-sounding difficulties that the clinician (or administrator) faces in putting results into practice. In addition, work with practical implications that is carried out in this way is much more likely to find general acceptance by the providers and users of the service concerned than where the epidemiologist has gone it alone, as he often can and has.

Will epidemiology meet its challenges and opportunities, and what are these?

Clearing the undergrowth

Fortunately, epidemiology is not by nature a field in which much effort has ever been devoted to abstruse problems of only academic interest; it is a practical discipline for which the labels 'pure' and 'applied' are mostly inappropriate, though sometimes used as a matter of convenience. Consequently, recent alterations in the organization of medical research not only left epidemiology largely unscathed, but actually improved its position, relatively if not also absolutely. Views expressed by medical research workers, including epidemiologists, on the White Paper (9) were mostly hostile, but at the end of the day the main principle underlying the New Deal, that value for money in research and development means results of a practical nature for the service concerned, was bound to favour disciplines such as epidemiology. (Some concern remains, however, over the implications of the arrangements for more basic subjects on which some aspects of epidemiology will increasingly depend.) The worsening economic climate of the last five years has also tended to favour work from which early developments and applications are likely, at the expense of work from which such returns cannot so easily be anticipated. 'Health services research', especially, has grown rapidly (32). In retrospect, the health departments' entry into research must be judged a success; with surprisingly little administrative overload and a willingness to take chances, they established the health services field as one of real potential benefit to the NHS, and as a rewarding one for the research worker. The departments' customer, or user, interests are now formally integrated into their research and development programmes; this was clearly necessary, but it will be a pity if the newly enlarged administrative research machinery (diagramatic representations of which will fill anyone daunted by transistor circuits with new hope) stifles the positive aspects of its largely *ad hoc* forerunner. These changes would have been needed sooner or later—their success may depend largely on their flexibility.

One inevitable consequence of the reorganization of medical research is the new jargon. Through the universities and their own research establishments, the health departments are now responsible for 'health services research', the MRC for the 'biomedical'. On any view, epidemiology straddles the shifting boundary between the two. The distinction probably has to be accepted for administrative purposes; provided this division of responsibility does not interfere with the natural flow of epidemiological inquiry from one side of it to the other, along the lines discussed earlier, the terminology may turn out to be no more than an irritation. But if the division becomes an obstacle, if the 'word-salad of jargon, incomprehensible to those not in the business' (see reference 8, discussing community medicine) divides epidemiologists into two groups, real damage will have been done, and ground lost.

In health services research particularly, the epidemiologist needs to be worldly wise in initiating his own work or responding to requests from others. First, he must ensure that what he is asked to do is researchable; many pressing issues either are not, or are posed in an unanswerable form, or call for methods that are too complex and impractical to make useful conclusions reasonably likely. Measuring 'quality of life' is probably a good example of the latter (considered again later). Next, a rather prevalent impression used to be that if the relevant research could be done, its results would almost certainly be put into practice; instances in which important decisions were taken before commissioned work was complete, however, demonstrate the fallacy of this assumption. Political motives, the pressure of public opinion, the urgency of many problems which demand immediate action, and situations where decisions can be made on commonsense grounds are probably the basis for change or for the *status quo* as often as the rational weighing-up of research findings. The reorganization of the NHS itself is a topical example of a change not conspicuous for prior research; not that any research would necessarily have been desirable or helpful. It is also probably naïve to assume that even where research has been requested and satisfactorily concluded, results will automatically be implemented even if these seem to offer an improvement on the existing state of affairs; other services may have higher priority. Finally, the extent to which the NHS can accommodate even changes of proven value is limited, probably very considerably, by its existing commitments.

How far those who do health services research should be involved in implementing their results is currently being debated. One view is that the research worker's responsibilities may often be on more than to answer certain limited questions, and that it is then up to others to decide what to do. On the other hand, it is obvious that those who have helped unravel the earlier parts of a problem will often want to be involved in putting their findings into practice. Research on health services covers a wide and rather amorphous area of contrasting activities, ranging from the clinical to the managerial. It is not even open to most epidemiologists to implement the results of a clinical trial of, say, place of treatment following myocardial infarction (31); this will mainly be a matter for their clinical colleagues. By contrast, the introduction and use of an information system that he has developed for a health authority is something the epidemiologist can hardly avoid. In fact, research will often imply implementation. If the epidemiologist has planned his inquiries with the clinicians or administrators concerned, and has ensured that the work is carried out and the results presented with due attention paid to local circumstances, the transition from his research to their service may be hard to define. For work on the mentally handicapped (29) and on the community hospital (5) services had to be set up or modified in order that the research objectives could be met. So long as the epidemiologist realizes that he has no absolute right to inflict his involvement in implementation on those who may not want it, careful project planning and the specific situation should usually make the extent of his useful service role apparent.

Health services research and development[1]

Earlier, the case was made for regarding epidemiology as a technique for answering many different sorts of questions, and for not attempting the precise definition of these questions as 'biochemical' or to do with 'health services'. Reluctantly, however, some kind of classification has to be made for further discussion.

It is not necessary to have a detailed knowledge of the history of medicine or the NHS to appreciate the main problems that the Service faces. Revolutionary advances in the diagnosis and treatment of some conditions, complete lack of progress in others (usually associated with multiple treatment methods, mostly of little or no value, but hallowed by tradition), the ageing population, staff shortages, the many professions in modern medicine, and until fairly recently, *ad hoc* administrative and management methods, are some (though by no means all) of the ingredients of the present situation. Demands for health services far exceed supply; resources are limited; there are no clear or generally agreed guidelines for deciding priorities; in many instances we have only the haziest notions about outcome, and therefore about the effectiveness of what we do. Despair of ever being able to improve matters would be an understandable reaction, and is, indeed, embodied in prophesies of the 'imminent collapse' of the NHS that have been made sporadically for almost as long as the Service has been in existence, though now with increasing frequency. A more optimistic view, however, is justified. The NHS is almost without rival in economically developed countries; its outstanding feature is not that it has shortcomings, but its achievement in making comprehensive care (of variable standards, certainly) available in almost all eventualities, and for virtually the entire population. The question is how the Service can be improved, within the constraints imposed on it. Can activities that

1. The NHS faces a series of unprecedented crises which are, at the time of writing, largely unresolved. It is assumed, and seems likely, that the aftermath of present difficulties will find the general structure and responsibilities of the country's health services unaltered, but the outcome of current problems cannot be predicted with certainty.

are not effective be identified, and can the resources involved be put to better use elsewhere? What steps can be taken to rectify undoubted deficiencies: in the care of the mentally handicapped, in reducing surgical waiting-lists, in the earlier detection of treatable disease, and so on? It is not enough to answer, as many do, that more and more money will solve these questions. Comparing proportions of Gross National Product allocated to various sectors by different countries is a popular pastime which, if it were the basis for decisions in this country, would probably result in substantially increased health expenditure. But increased financial input is no guarantee of improved health and health care standards, and there are other demands to be considered; whether health is more or less important than education, housing, or a reliable train service is a value judgement that the community has to make as a whole. No special group should expect to be able to impose its own values on others. As well as pressing for further resources where these are necessary, medicine has an equal duty to ensure that it is making effective use of those it already has. Some wastage in an undertaking of the size and complexity of the NHS is inevitable, but this is no reason to avoid attempting to reduce it as far as possible.

Provided, once again, that he chooses carefully, the epidemiologist clearly has a leading role to play. Faced with the numerous and varied questions needing study, he may be tempted to 'attempt global answers to global problems, mainly on the grounds that the value of health services as a whole is what is under study, and that the piecemeal study of individual problems is too time-consuming' (30). This is, however, probably the wrong strategy, for reasons to do mainly with the difficulty of measuring outcome.

Likely to be of greater value than general studies of health services as a whole are carefully selected and executed evaluative studies of single issues. The case for this kind of work, especially by randomized controlled trials, has been particularly advocated by Cochrane (12). Place of treatment, length of stay in hospital, type of treatment, and the value of laboratory investigations are some of the questions requiring and open to investigation. A good illustration of work of this sort on the place of treatment following myocardial infarction (31), not only demonstrated that hospital was not necessarily the place of choice (Table

1), but also (and perhaps more importantly) that trials of this kind are necessary, practicable, and ethical.

TABLE 1

Mortality in a randomized controlled trial of place of treatment for myocardial infarction

Place of treatment allocated	*Treated at home*		*Treated in hospital*	
	No.	*Mortality* %	*No.*	*Mortality* %
At random	174	9·8	169	14·2
Electively	106	11·3	754	16·8

Source: Reference 31.

One of Cochrane's examples illustrates well the need, so often overlooked, to study how knowledge gained may best be put into practice. The advent of effective chemotherapy for tuberculosis led to a series of inquiries on its efficient clinical application. Place of treatment was investigated, notably in Madras, and it became clear that in-patient treatment, with its accompanying prolonged bed-rest, was no more effective than out-patient management. Mean length of hospital stay in this country for patients with respiratory tuberculosis fell very slowly, however, for many years after this information was available, and Cochrane suggests that the optimum approach to the treatment of pulmonary tuberculosis is still not entirely clear, though chemotherapy has now been to hand for a considerable time.

Effectiveness and efficiency, or lack of them, can also be demonstrated by observational methods. In one study of the value of intravenous urography in the investigation of hypertension, the effects of the procedure on subsequent clinical management were recorded (1); in another the role of other, less costly, tests was considered (28). Each linked radiological data with other data in the case-notes, and each indicated the limited value of urography. Nevertheless, there is little doubt that the clinical trial is one of the epidemiologist's most powerful methods, and that it can be successfully applied to situations beyond its traditional use in the evaluation of medicines, and hardly considered only a few years ago.

Health services research poses certain problems for the epidemiologist over and above those already considered, and of a sort that tend to be swept under the carpet. First, there is the question of time-scale. The epidemiologist generally ought not to be encouraged to work if a decision on the topic in question is to be made before the work is complete. Equally, however, he cannot expect important decisions to be deferred, perhaps for several years, while he carries out studies that are often, in the nature of things, long-term. He has two main choices; one is to concede that his particular skills are not appropriate, and that others should be used. The second may be to omit some of the preliminary steps he might otherwise take over methods to be used, and to make other sacrifices in the interests of speed. There may, for example, be a case for self-validating measures which, if positive results emerge in the shape of clear differences between groups, can probably be interpreted at their face value. In fact, many of the indices of cigarette smoking (for example, even the number smoked per day; the 'drooping cigarette' habit, a phrase coined by Brett and Benjamin (7) to describe a particular way of smoking that is associated with an increased lung cancer mortality) have never, strictly speaking, been validated, or have only been validated in retrospect. The situation is very different, however, in trying to assess return to health in an elderly stroke patient, where it may be far from clear that a method claimed to measure functional improvement actually does so. There may indeed sometimes be a case for speed at the expense of thoroughness, but cutting corners in epidemiology is notoriously risky; it is certainly not the conventional wisdom of academic social medicine. Chances may occasionally have to be taken, though, and accepted by customer and contractor alike. One obvious safeguard is to ask and attempt to answer only one question at a time. It is astonishing how difficult this can be; the basically simple clinical trial can very soon become a complex and potentially unmanageable 'fishing expedition', as different measurements are added in attempts to study the associations and causes of the condition, as well as to compare methods of treating it. Over the next few years, epidemiology applied to health services research must confront these issues.

Epidemiology and other disciplines

Operational research (OR) is being increasingly used in health services research where the protracted time-scale of epidemiology causes difficulties. For the newcomer to the subject, there seem to be as many definitions of OR as there are of epidemiology; essentially, OR in health services research uses model-building in order to make predictions as a possible basis for policy; and since the models require data for their construction and manipulation, there are obviously many ways in which OR and epidemiology overlap. A good example concerns screening for carcinoma of the cervix. How often women should be screened, which groups should receive special attention, and the implications of different policies for the relevant services could be examined by a combination of prospective observational studies and clinical trials; but these would obviously be expensive and time-consuming. An alternative approach (see reference 26, for example) is to use data that are available (for example, on mortality and the acceptability of tests) in a simulation model, which may also have to include assumptions about points on which there is little or no information. The consequences of different policies can then be compared. Naturally, the quality of the results will depend on the quality of the data used, and the extent to which the assumptions made are realistic; so that simulation is not an automatic panacea. Another example, and one for which a model is almost essential, is in estimating the number of beds necessary in an intensive therapy unit (47). From data which established how many patients could be expected to need intensive care at any time, the relationship between beds provided and the probability of turning patients away could be established. Another example arises with length of stay in hospital; this can almost certainly be reduced (even further than has already occurred) for many conditions, and this is often invoked as a means of reducing or abolishing waiting-lists. But what will be the effects of increased turnover on surgical teams, for example, and on the demand for theatre and anaesthetists' time, and on nursing staff? Models are likely to help in deciding whether, and if so how, further potential reductions in length of stay can best be realized.

Epidemiology has so far had a rather disappointing and unfruitful relationship with *sociology* (though there are some notable exceptions, many of which are in the field of reproductive biology). The notion that there are social elements in determining the onset of disease, reactions to illness, and demands for care, is, of course, not new, and is reflected in 'social medicine'. The public health reforms of the last century and subsequent differential social class improvements in mortality and infant mortality demonstrated what common-sense would have predicted. The value of social class as a general index has been repeatedly tested and proved but, while it obviously embodies sociological features, it is too general in its construction and use to be considered to reflect only the latter.

The crystallization of social medicine from a number of more or less vague origins into a defined specialty was largely the achievement of Professor J. A. Ryle, for many years a practising physician at Guy's Hospital, and briefly Regius Professor of Physic at Cambridge, before becoming the first Professor of Social Medicine at Oxford. His accounts of the content and purpose of the subject are as apt today as they were thirty years ago (44, 45); they set a syllabus that would be hard to quarrel with seriously, some of which has been met where the aetiology and prevention of many diseases are concerned. Social medicine deals with health and disease, in individuals as well as in groups, through a number of disciplines: epidemiology, medical statistics, the social sciences, operational research, and management and administration. How far has sociological investigation contributed? If ever there was a challenge tailor-made for the sociologist in medicine, a touchstone by which to prove himself, it is provided by cigarette smoking. As the role of cigarettes in lung cancer and other diseases become clearer, so did the need for studies of the motives for smoking, of the difficulties of dropping the habit and of ways of communicating with smokers. Hopes were pinned on health education to be planned in accordance with knowledge gained. Yet failure has been almost total. Awareness of the consequences of smoking is virtually universal, but the most recent signs are of increases, not decreases, in cigarette consumption. Table 2 gives food for thought. Is it really correct to assume, as it usually is, that the 45-year-old man who smokes 15 cigarettes a day would be very concerned to know that his life expectancy is five years less than the twenty-five years he might otherwise expect? Does information of this sort mean anything at all to the 25- or 15-year-old smoker, and if not, could it be made to? In fact, it seems that the smoking public has, perhaps largely unconsciously, assessed the odds in the form in which they have been presented and found them

TABLE 2

Life expectancy for American men at various ages who smoke 10–19 cigarettes per day, compared with men who do not smoke

Cigarettes per day	*Present age (years)* 25	35	45	55	65
0	48·6	39·2	30·0	21·4	14·1
10–19	43·1	33·8	25·0	17·4	11·2

Source: Royal College of Physicians Report, *Smoking and Health Now* (1971).

acceptable. None of these questions is a defence of cigarette smoking; but have the right questions been asked in the right way? To take another example, are the difficulties of persuading the high-risk, low social class woman to accept screening for cervical cancer really amenable to fruitful inquiry along the lines adopted so far? What people say are their views and intentions in health matters on the one hand, and what they actually do on the other, are often too discrepant for policies to be based on the former, popular though such approaches are. None the less, the conviction that there is much more than gold at the end of the rainbow to be had from sociology in health care is a real one. The relative imprecision of many of the indices of social behaviour and social change, and the importance of factors determining illness and reactions to it (housing and education, for example) that are outside the training and direct professional concern of most doctors are challenges to the epidemiologist and sociologist alike (49).

In some ways, it is puzzling that epidemiologists did not turn to *economists* for help a good deal earlier than they actually did. Yet it was not so very long ago that, by and large, medicine was provided with what it said it needed, so that, on the definition of economics as the allocation of *scarce* resources (37), health economics may not then have had the relevance and sense of urgency it has now. Perhaps the event which clearly symbolized the end of the era of comparative plenty in this country was the discouragement, amounting almost to a ban, of heart transplantation. It is a fact, however unpalatable, that we simply cannot do everything in the health field we should like to do: though there are still many heads in the sand. Measurements of effectiveness are one expression of the increasing constraints under which the

NHS has to operate; and these constraints are not all necessarily bad. Talk of medical audit and the introduction of programme-budgeting are other expressions. Some of these applications of economics are not the direct concern of the epidemiologist in health services research, but call for his skills in providing the information on which they are based.

In technical terms, 'positive' economics deals with how the economic system works, and the influence of changes within the system. Again, smoking provides an apt example. For years, argument about the net economic effects of smoking has rumbled on, unresolved; it is not wholly academic, by any means. The Royal College of Physicians report *Smoking and Health Now* (40), gave new impetus to the topic, resulting in a general survey by an interdepartmental government inquiry (13). The subject is very complex; there is no single answer to the question, but many, depending on the viewpoint adopted (2). Pensions, earnings, the age structure of the population, the nature and possibly the quantity of sickness, and medical manpower requirements could all be influenced by the decline in cigarette smoking that most hope to see. There is therefore good reason to try to clarify what the effects of such a decline (or of an increase, which in women is a serious reality) would be.

Implicit in this sort of work on smoking, though not the main reason for it, is the opportunity to choose between different possible courses of action. 'Normative' economics is explicitly concerned with the formulation and choice of policies. For example, different methods of achieving the same objective may incur substantially different costs. In studies on the treatment of varicose veins, Chant and his colleagues (10) showed that the outcome following injection/compression sclerotherapy was little different, in terms of re-treatment needed in the next three years, from surgical treatment; patients preferred the former. When the costs of the two methods were compared (36), however, it was clear that injection/compression sclerotherapy was less costly than surgery to both the NHS and the patient (judged in the latter case by a comparison of loss of earnings). Few would quarrel with the potential value of this application of economics.

Policy is also at the centre of another but controversial area of mutual concern to the epidemiologist and the health economist. Since we cannot afford everything we need, priorities have to be established between competing claims by politicians, administrators, and the community as a whole, whose concern they are and will remain. Decisions in this context, as in any other, are likely to be more rational, or at least defensible, if they are informed. Epidemiologists and health economists will not suggest that because a district geriatric service costs less than one for mental handicap, the former should be chosen. They would, in the present state of the art, have to be very cautious about doing so even if they wished to, because of the difficulties of measuring outcome. To be able to say something about the likely costs and consequences of the two services, however, even in approximate terms, is likely to be as helpful as the provision of different types of information for other aspects of health care.

Nevertheless, support for the cost-benefit approach to health services is still limited in many (including some epidemiological) quarters. For instance, and to return again to smoking, it has been argued that it is largely irrelevant whether smoking-related disease decreases as a result of changing smoking habits, since those with other conditions will still need and demand medical services. Resources freed by a decline in cigarette consumption, the argument goes, will be more than swallowed up by these hitherto unmet demands. Why therefore attempt to predict changes in smoking-related diseases? There are several answers. First, and most important, treatment of hitherto unmet demand in itself implies a benefit that could not previously be conferred. Secondly, money saved in health services does not have to be spent on them. There are opportunity costs of the (largely ineffective) treatment of lung cancer without, as well as within, the NHS. The extent to which resources saved in one area of health services were used in another area, or outside the health field altogether, would give some indication of society's valuation of the benefits derived from the savings. (Fein [18] and Glass [19] have given balanced accounts of the pros and cons of cost-effectiveness and cost-benefit analyses in health services.) Thirdly, alterations in the burden of some specific diseases could have major health service consequences; a substantial decline in the incidence of lung cancer would, for example, have obvious effects on chest surgery as a specialty, and it would be foolish not to have considered the consequences of these and other effects in good time.

A rather different use of economics that may involve the epidemiologist is in assessing different ways of paying for medical care. On the face of it, a fee-for-service basis may encourage the doctor to over-investigate and overtreat, whereas capitation systems are less likely to do so. Much has been written on this subject, a high proportion rather theoretical in nature, but a good illustration of how the epidemiologist and the economist may usefully collaborate is the comparison of operation rates in Canada and in England and Wales, made by Vayda (50). This showed rates nearly twice as high in Canada as in England and Wales, with substantially higher operative mortality in the former than the latter. One suggested explanation for these findings (clearly not to be accepted uncritically, but equally clearly well worth further study) are differences in the organization of and payment for health services. Inquiries of this sort have real potential for making a practical impact, perhaps mainly in countries where there are possibilities for radical alterations in the way health care is provided and financed.

The control of smoking may yet turn out to be achieved largely by the implications of economic analyses. A current controversy on the price elasticity of demand for tobacco goods is unresolved (3, 4, 41) but illustrates very well the importance of developing and applying the appropriate techniques.

Other uses of economics in health services are more the domain of the economist on his own, or in conjunction with the administrator, but it is clear that the economist and epidemiologist should collaborate on appropriate occasions. To the epidemiologist, the economist brings unfamiliar but powerful new methods to bear; often, the epidemiologist will be no more than the technician, providing the necessary data. On other occasions, however, it will be the epidemiologist who formulates the hypothesis and calls upon the economist for what will eventually, one hopes, be routine assistance. What has to be avoided is the doctor grappling with the complexities of modern health economics on the back of an envelope, or the economist, both feet firmly in the air, advocating health policies that are unrealistic or impossible; both occur.

Collaboration between the epidemiologist and the economist is at the start of a difficult but probably very rewarding course. There is still a great deal to be done on basic methods as well as on defining what the subject may or may not be able to achieve.

'It is a field in which gardening is real and botany is bogus' (14), but there is plenty of gardening to be done. Whether the applications of health economics that have been discussed will be of practical use has become a matter of study and experiment rather than speculation.

Administrators belong to a service, rather than a research, discipline with which many epidemiologists are concerned. Most contacts are over the design of studies the latter are to carry out on behalf of, rather than with, the former, and over the implementation of results. There is, however, one obvious area in which investigative collaboration is increasingly needed, and that is in the collection, analysis, and interpretation of information. Like the multidisciplinary team, health services information runs the risk of becoming something of an end in itself. The need for digestible information of the right sort is obvious, but solving the familiar problem of turning information into knowledge is not easy. Workable proposals on information systems in the integrated NHS have been made by Knox and his colleagues (27), but unworkable proposals, as often the expression of real enthusiasm as of anything else, could make excessively heavy demands on skills that are hard to come by.

The *statistician*'s contribution will be as much an essential part of epidemiology in the future as it has been in the past. By now, the epidemiologist should feel secure enough to ask himself, occasionally, how much of the time he occupies the driver's seat.

Measuring outcome

The difficulty of defining and using appropriate measures of what has been achieved as a result of treatment or the introduction of a service has already arisen several times; it provides present and future epidemiology with one of its main challenges. Many have come to grief attempting solutions to the problem.

Mortality data are easy to come by, and valuable in spite of their acknowledged shortcomings. With rather few exceptions, however, readily available morbidity data covering all sections of the population are few and far between. Data on the use of services still depend mainly on unlinked systems such as the *Hospital In-Patient Enquiry*, and there are signs of restlessness over the early but largely unfulfilled promises of Hospital Activity Analysis as a means of overcoming this deficiency. But even linked data on contacts with health services would leave 'quality of life' unmeasured. While there is wide agreement over the theoretical relevance of indices of this type, efforts to establish them have not really succeeded, at least in terms of measures that could be agreed and put to practical, on-going use. A number of preliminary attempts have been made (6, 11, 17, 39); the measures suggested may have some value in *ad hoc* situations, but hardly routinely.

What, then, can be made of the indices that are generally available? First, the value of mortality data should not be overlooked, even if death may not be the most appropriate measure of outcome. Doll (14) has shown how changes in death-rates may give valuable indications on the effectiveness of care in hypertension, gall-bladder disease, appendicitis, asthma, prostatic hyperplasia, and abortion (thus providing another illustration that the clinical trial is not always a *sine qua non* of evaluation in health care). Secondly, expanded record-linkage systems (subject to the satisfactory solution of the confidentiality issues involved) and use of inquiries like the General Household Survey could give better quality morbidity data than we have at present.

Prevention

While health services research now offers the epidemiologist almost unlimited opportunities, the fact remains that many of the latter are based on the cure and care consequences of failures to prevent. Contemporary health expectations are overshadowed by arterial and chronic respiratory disease: whether measured by mortality, sickness absence from work, or by other indices (33). Death from lung cancer, and disability from locomotor disease and mental disorder indicate other major unprevented conditions.

Clinically manifest arterial disease, especially ischaemic heart disease, almost certainly poses the largest and probably the most intractable medical problem in economically developed countries. It has taken over twenty years of one of epidemiology's most costly enterprises to establish a modest capacity to predict onset, to realize that, in practical terms, secondary prevention is difficult, perhaps almost to the point of being unattainable, and for several countries to advocate measures for primary prevention that are of unproven value and low acceptability. In this country, death-rates from ischaemic heart disease in middle-aged men continue to rise.

That diseases can be prevented without precise knowledge of their causes should never be overlooked. However, when long-term effort of the order devoted to arterial disease has been spent for so little return, the signs are either that the disease cannot be prevented, or that very detailed studies of its aetiology and of possible methods of modifying disordered function are necessary. Fundamental questions have barely been asked. What is the real relationship of atheroma to clinical disease, and with which are we primarily concerned? What are the epidemiological differences, as well as similarities, between the various manifestations of arterial disease at various sites? How far and how quickly can the epidemiologist look beyond traditional confines, to increasingly detailed studies of lipid metabolism, to minerals and trace elements, and the role of the haemostatic system? Is it necessary to resolve the century-old controversy on the aetiology of atheroma, and if so, can this be assisted by epidemiological methods? In approaching these questions, it would be short-sighted of the epidemiologist not to make it his business actively to stimulate modern technology in the relevant fields to meet his needs, let alone neglect technical developments already available but unexploited. Growing interest in carbon monoxide, as a marker of the extent to which the gaseous phase of tobacco smoke is inhaled, and perhaps as a specific factor in the development of atheroma, may enable the more accurate prediction than hitherto of those at risk of smoking-related disease. Information of this sort, coupled with new ideas on potentially safer smoking habits (42) and with possible biochemical methods of identifying smokers at special risk (25) may prove to be yet another way, not really envisaged even quite recently, of approaching the smoking problem. Biochemical and microbiological analyses of the faeces (23) combined with dietary studies in prospective field surveys may well go far towards establishing the causes of large bowel cancer. The maximum exploitation of these and similar developments will depend to a greater or lesser degree on how epidemiology and laboratory disciplines respond to the challenges and opportunities they present to one another. The short-term returns on aetiological studies may not, over-all, be obvious, but the potential for rapid, even spectacular, advances certainly exists, and must not be overlooked as a result of preoccupation with apparently more immediate issues.

Many community physicians have responsibilities for environmental health matters. This is an exciting and growing field of interest for the epidemiologist, and in its widest sense involves concern with industrial hazards, the unwanted effects of medicines, the safety of foods and so on (20). With experience already gained (from the delay in recognizing the effects of thalidomide in pregnancy, for example) the early detection and modification of environmental health hazards is another way in which prevention may often be able to forestall demands for care. But the epidemiologist working in this area will have to assume increasing responsibility for data and advice on how to strike a balance between costs and benefits, both clinical and social. Hardly a month now passes without evidence being presented that appears to incriminate a medicine, a food, or a chemical in common use. The appropriate course of action over an industrial hazard, where workers' safety is paramount, and only a relatively small part of the whole population is exposed, is often much easier to identify and pursue than over the possible ill-effects of tea, coffee, potatoes, and many other dietary items, for example, which are part and parcel of everyday life for most people, or of self-medication. Conflicting expert views, held in good faith and usually no more than an expression of real scientific doubts, can be misinterpreted as scaremongering if risks eventually turn out to have been overestimated, or as complacency if the hazard is confirmed. It is possible to be too cautious, as well as too optimistic about safety; in 'Amphotericin Pharmacophobia' Symmers (48) described five cases in which patients died as a result of the withholding of amphotericin, although the preparation was clearly indicated. As the epidemiology of the environment develops, staying on the tightrope all the time will become increasingly difficult; the trick will be not to fall off too often.

Screening

Nearly all the themes discussed so far (priorities, evaluation of services, cost-benefit, prevention, the contribution of technology) come together in screening. This complex approach to the early detection, treatment, and prevention of disease is, of course, very much the epidemiologist's territory. The subject has been dealt with in detail by many authorities; here, only some general points are considered.

Epidemiology is the study of health and disease in human populations and, traditionally, its applications have also been thought of in terms of the well-being of groups or communities, rather than of the individual. Prescriptive screening hardly fits in with this view; it certainly depends on epidemiological assessments for its initiation and implementation, but is, in practice, very much directed towards the individual. Nothing perhaps could be more personal than information about possible developmental abnormalities that perinatal screening methods are now making increasingly available. Epidemiologists are therefore equally concerned with the health of individuals as well as of groups, and they restrict their horizons if they insist otherwise. Ryle (43) regarded 'social medicine (for all its needful associations with public hygiene) as a logical development from and a direct expansion of clinical medicine'. There is, he claimed, 'no sharp division between individual and social medicine'. Another perspective with the same conclusion comes from the case for screening in general practice put forward by Hart (21). 'Effective and genuinely continuous personal care will depend more and more on recorded data designed for rapid future retrieval, obtained on a basis of screening.' Screening in 'patient-orientated anticipatory care' calls for new research initiatives, and further adds to the responsibilities as well as the opportunities of the epidemiologist.

Epidemiology overseas

All stand to gain by the contribution that epidemiology can make to research and development in the Third World. First, international disease comparisons have already done much for the study of aetiology and there are still many unexploited opportunities. Secondly, there are some research projects where the opportunities in the field can only be exploited if experienced epidemiological, statistical, and computing help can be provided: as they often can by centres in countries where these disciplines are well established. Leprosy, for example, is a disease which still causes a huge burden of chronic disability and deformity in the world's endemic areas, where prevalence figures of 3 per cent, and often more, are not unusual. For various reasons, mainly because many factors besides *Mycobacterium leprae* appear to determine clinical onset, leprosy is particularly suitable for study by epidemiological methods; but large populations and information on many factors are needed.

Thirdly, the rudimentary nature of health services in many countries overseas provides opportunities for study and experiment that can benefit both those countries and others with more developed health services. It is only necessary to see the skill with which paramedical assistants can deal with complex clinical situations in which medical supervision is limited or nonexistent, to realize how inappropriate the division of labour within the NHS often is. There is little doubt that a great deal of medical time could be freed by increased professional willingness to allow others to do jobs that doctors presently regard as unsuitable for delegation: and so on, between nurses and ward assistants, remedial therapists and voluntary workers. There is probably no group within a district general hospital, for example, whose work could not be made more interesting in this way; is it too optimistic to believe that standards of care might also rise as a result? In the context of current inflation and the scarcity of nearly all resources, the NHS and all who work in it will have to be ready to take a leaf out of the overseas book, and realize that ingenuity and imagination, as well as cash, are needed. There is a strong case to be made for the contention that every epidemiology or health care team in this country primarily engaged in research should seek some involvement in work in the 'under-doctored disease-ridden bush' (38).

Conclusion

There is much more epidemiological work to be done than there are epidemiologists to do it (another reason, incidentally, for the importance of selecting researchable subjects with some likelihood of useful and practical results, and also for further encouraging the active participation of those who do not think of themselves as epidemiologists in population-based research). In general, career prospects in epidemiology could hardly be better than they presently are, though some important details of career structure still have to be settled. The establishment of the Faculty of Community Medicine and of its examination for membership, together with the recommendations of the Hunter Working Party (24) on the community physician have already encouraged active project participation as the training method of choice in epidemiology; classroom teaching can too easily make it dull. The deep end is undoubtedly the one in which to learn the subject, since epidemiology is based on common sense and attention to detail, not on the mastery of a highly technical laboratory discipline; at the same time, the student has the satisfaction of contributing to work of practical value which might otherwise not be done.

Epidemiology already has many considerable achievements to its name as it enters what may be a Golden Age of opportunity; it is assured of continued active encouragement, and, relatively at least, of generous support. But: 'unto whomsoever much is given, of him shall be much required; and to whom men have committed much, of him they will ask the more' (Luke 12:48): the moral, aptly enough, of the parable of the faithful servants.

REFERENCES

1. Atkinson, A. B., and Kellett, R. J. (1974). *Jl R. Coll. Physic.* 8, 175.
2. Atkinson, A. B., and Meade, T. W. (1974). *Jl R. Statist. Soc.* Series A, 137, 297.
3. —— Skegg, J. L. (1973). In: *Manchester School* (September edition).
4. —— —— (1974). *Br. J. prev. soc. Med.* 28, 45.
5. Bennett, A. E. (1974). In McLachlan, G. (ed.), *Positions, Movements, and Directions in Health Services Research* (Oxford University Press for the Nuffield Provincial Hospitals Trust).
6. Breslow, L. (1972). *Internat. J. Epidemiol.* 1, 347.
7. Brett, G. Z., and Benjamin, B. (1968). *Br. med. J.* 3, 82.
8. *Br. med. J.* 2 (1974), 186.
9. Central Policy Review Staff (1972). *Framework for Government Research and Development* (Cmnd. 5046) (London: HMSO).
10. Chant, A. D. B., Jones, H. O., and Weddell, J. M. (1972). *Lancet*, ii, 1188.
11. Chiang, C. L., and Cohen, R. D., (1973). *Internat. J. Epidemiol.* 2, 7.
12. Cochrane, A. L. (1972). *Effectiveness and Efficiency. Random Reflections on Health Services.* Rock Carling Monograph (London: Nuffield Provincial Hospitals Trust).
13. Department of Health and Social Security (1972). *Smoking and Health* (London: HMSO).

14. DOLL, R. (1973). *Proc. R. Soc. Med.*
15. —— HILL, A. B. (1954). *Br. med. J.* 1, 1451.
16. —— —— (1964). Ibid. 1, 1399 and 1460.
17. FANSHEL, S. (1972). *Internat. J. Epidemiol.* 1, 319.
18. FEIN, R. (1970). In McLachlan, G., and McKeown, T. (eds), *Medical History and Medical Care* (Oxford University Press for the Nuffield Provincial Hospitals Trust).
19. GLASS, N. J. (1973). *Hlth Trends*, 5, 51.
20. GODBER, G. E. (1973). In McLachlan, G. (ed.), *The Future—and Present Indicatives, Problems and Progress in Medical Care*, Ninth Series (Oxford University Press for the Nuffield Provincial Hospitals Trust).
21. HART, J. T. (1974). *Update*, 8, 981.
22. HILL, A. B. (1965). *Proc. R. Soc. Med.* 58, 295.
23. HILL, M. J., CROWTHER, J. S., DRASAR, B. S., HAWKSWORTH, G., ARIES, V., and WILLIAMS, R. E. O. (1971). *Lancet*, i, 95.
24. HUNTER, R. B. (1972). *Report of the Working Party on Medical Administrators* (London: HMSO).
25. KELLERMAN, G., SHAW, C. R., and LUYTEN-KELLERMAN, M. (1973). *New Engl. J. Med.* 289, 934.
26. KNOX, E. G. (1973) In McLachlan, G. (ed.), *The Future—and Present Indicatives, Problems and Progress in Medical Care*, Ninth Series (Oxford University Press for the Nuffield Provincial Hospitals Trust).
27. —— MORRIS, J. N., and HOLLAND, W. W. (1972). *Lancet*, ii, 696.
28. KREEL, L. ELTON, A. HABERSHON, R., MASON, A. M. S., and MEADE, T. W. (1974). *Br. med. J.* (4,3).
29. KUSHLICK, A. (1974). In McLachlan, G. (ed.), *Positions, Movements, and Directions in Health Services Research* (Oxford University Press for the Nuffield Provincial Hospitals Trust).
30. *Lancet*, i (1973), 1293.
31. MATHER, H. G., PEARSON, W. G., READ, K. L. Q., SHAW, D. B., STEED, G. R., THORNE, M. G., JONES, S., GUERRIER, C. J., ERANT, C. D., MCHUGH, P. M., CHOWDHURY, N. R., JAFARY, M. H., and WALLACE, T. J. (1971). *Br. med. J.* 3, 334.
32. MCLACHLAN, G. (ed.) (1973) *Portfolio for Health 2, Problems and Progress in Medical Care*, Eighth Series (Oxford University Press for the Nuffield Provincial Hospitals Trust).
33. MEADE, T. W. (1974) In *Population and the New Biology* (New York: Academic Press.
34. MORRIS, J. N. (1970). *Uses of Epidemiology* (London: Livingstone).
35. *Nature*, 245 (1973), 61.
36. PIACHAUD, D., and WEDDELL, J. M. (1972). *Lancet*, ii, 1191.
37. ROBBINS, L. (1932). *An Essay on the Nature and Significance of Economic Science* (London: Macmillan).

38. ROSENHEIM, M. (1968). *Lancet*, ii, 821.

39. ROSSER, R. M. and WATTS, V. C. (1972). *Internat. J. Epidemiol.* 1, 361.

40. ROYAL COLLEGE OF PHYSICIANS (1971). *Smoking and Health Now* (London: Pitman).

41. RUSSELL, M. A. H. (1973). *Br. J. prev. Soc. Med.* 27, 1.

42. —— (1974). *Lancet*, i, 254.

43. RYLE, J. A. (1943). *Br. med. J.* 2, 634.

44. —— (1945). *Br. J. Indust. Med.* 2, 108.

45. —— (1948). *Practitioner*, 161, 5.

46. SHAPIRO, S., STRAX, P., and VENET, L. (1971). *J. Am. med. Ass.* 215 1777.

47. STRINGER, J. (1970). In *Resources in Medicine* (King Edward's Hospital Fund for London).

48. SYMMERS, W. ST. C. (1973). *Br. med. J.* 4, 460.

49. TOWNSEND, P. (1974). *Lancet*, i, 1179.

50. VAYDA, E. (1973). *New Engl. J. Med.* 289, 1224.